As Nora Jo Fades Away

Confessions of a Caregiver

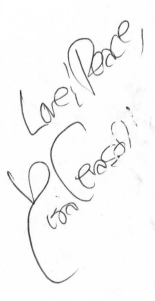

As Nora Jo Fades Away

Confessions of a Caregiver

Five Star Publications Inc.

Chandler, Arizona

Linda F. Radke, President
Five Star Publications, Inc.
PO Box 6698
Chandler, AZ 85246-6698
480-940-8182

www.AsNoraJoFadesAway.com

Library of Congress Cataloging-in-Publication Data

Cerasoli, Lisa, 1969-
  As Nora Jo fades away : confessions of a caregiver : a memoir / by Lisa
Cerasoli.
    p. cm.
  ISBN-13: 978-1-58985-190-0
  ISBN-10: 1-58985-190-0
1. Cerasoli, Nora Jo--Mental health. 2. Cerasoli, Lisa, 1969- 3. Alzheimer's
disease--Patients--Care. 4. Alzheimer's disease--Patients--United States--
Biography. 5. Caregivers--United States--Biography. I. Title.
  RC523.C435 2010
  362.196'8310092--dc22
  [B]
                                        2010003274

Printed in the United States of America

Editor: Paul Howey
Cover Design by Kris Taft Miller
Interior Design by Linda Longmire
Project Manager: Sue DeFabis

First Edition
10 9 8 7 6 5 4 3 2 1

The first thing that strikes you about Cerasoli's memoir is her steadfast refusal to manipulate us. Instead of tugging on our heartstrings to produce easy tears, she writes with a rigorous, clear-eyed lack of sentimentality and sly humor which only heightens the book's emotional impact. CONFESSIONS... is a passionate tribute to an unforgettable woman and a lesson in love under seemingly impossible circumstances.

Rob Potter, Story Analyst,
HBO and CASTLE ROCK ENTERTAINMENT

As seen in her previous work, "Confessions of a Caregiver" once again showcases Lisa Cerasoli's brilliant ability of weaving wit and warmth into grim subject matter. This memoir is a refreshing reflection of an inevitable human consideration: What would you do if faced with the responsibility of an aging loved one?

Bill Hinkle, Television Producer

Lisa Cerasoli immerses humor into a dark, frightening and lonely experience ... caring for someone you love as they are robbed of their mind and identity. This is a brave and honest account of her reluctant decision to become a caregiver and how it has changed her reality forever.

Jeannie (Messer) Leonard, Registered Nurse
Rush University Medical Center, Chicago, IL

This is an epidemic that people aren't facing. Cerasoli's portrayal of the challenges of taking care of her grandmother, Nora Jo proves that through wit, stark honesty and compassion it can be done. "In home" care is tough, but it's the best form of love and stability a family could give someone who's dying of Alzheimer's.

Laura Dupras, MSW

This story is honest without bias, desperately funny and a true heartbreaker. Keep it handy as a reminder of the genuine love we are all capable of.

Ruth Almén, Regional Director,
Upper Peninsula Region, Greater MI Chapter, Alzheimer's Association

As Nora Jo Fades Away
Confessions of a Caregiver

By Lisa Cerasoli

This book is fittingly dedicated to
A woman who's been
My Grandmother
Mentor
"Mother,"
BFF
Cooking coach
Drinking buddy
Partner in wit
Partner in grit
And who has now stepped into the role of my
beloved other daughter:

Nora Josephine Cerasoli

"You've been a steady bright light
in my roller coaster of a life.
And you've dished out more love than raviolis
(if that's even humanly possible)."

$\mathcal{A}$ $\mathcal{B}uck$ a $\mathcal{B}ook!$

One dollar for every book sold will go directly into a fund for the Alzheimer's Association and Leeza's Place.

To volunteer your time, make your own contribution or obtain more information check out your local Alzheimer's Association ... or get a hold of mine!

THE ALZHEIMER'S ASSOCIATION
800-272-3900 (National Helpline 24/7)

The Greater Michigan Chapter
906-228-3910
ruth.almen@alz.org (Regional Director)
phil.puotinen@alz.org (Wraparound Facilitator/Program Coordinator)
brenda.bickler@alz.org (Office Coordinator)

Or go to:

LEEZA'S PLACE "A Place for Caregivers"
www.leezasplace.org
1-888-655-3392 (1-888-OK-Leeza)

Leeza's Place is a community gathering and resource center for caregivers impacted by chronic or progressive illness offering connections, individual guidance, information and referrals, as well as a calendar full of programs to Educate, Empower & Energize.

Information including the locations of The Leeza Gibbons Memory Foundation and Leeza's Places located across the country can be found on the website. To send an email write to: info@leezasplace.org.

And introducing, My Caregiver's Wake Up Call ™
Lisa Cerasoli shares her care giving experiences with hope, humor and heart! Enjoy 30 Inspirational wake up calls set to beautiful music.

MY WAKE UP CALL™
Motivational Alarm Clock Messages
Awaken you each morning with positive energy!
www.mywakeupcalls.net
Download messages to MP3, iPhone, or purchase on CDs or buy the Alarm Clock.

DISCLAIMER

The stories I have spun
And the confessions that have been done
Have come with blessings from Above.

If some tales sound too bold,
This is how they have been retold.
They've molded my mind like hand to glove.

We all know that Time twists a memory
Into a shadow of what we knew it to be,
And that's okay. That's Life. That's Love.

DEFINITIONS

Alzheimer's Disease – A severe neurological disorder marked by progressive dementia.

Dementia – Irreversible deterioration of intellectual faculties with accompanying emotional disturbances. Madness. Insanity.

Insanity – A prolonged condition of mental disorder relieved intermittently by periods of clear-mindedness.

Memoir – An account of the personal experiences of an author. A biographical sketch, outline or informal story.

Memory – The mental faculty of retaining and recalling past experience.

Remember – To keep in mind as worthy of affection or recognition.

Source: The American Heritage Dictionary, Second College Edition

Foreword by Leeza Gibbons

I meet a lot of good people in my job as an interviewer. Many of them have something powerful to contribute and some do it with a unique approach. But I didn't expect what Lisa Cerasoli has to offer and it is precisely her ability to disarm that is her greatest weapon. Lisa embodies my axiom: "A Call to Action." Her father called her to say he was dying of cancer and asked if she would come home. Forty-eight hours later, Lisa boarded a plane to Michigan. She answered "that call" in 2003, leaving Hollywood and changing the course of her life and her purpose on this planet forever.

I believe we all wonder what we'd do if confronted by a moment of truth. Will we invest the emotional collateral to face it with grace? Lisa did. And her personal call to action didn't stop with her father's cancer. In 2008, her late father's mother, Nora Jo was diagnosed with advanced Alzheimer's disease. Lisa and her family immediately moved her in with them. That was two and a half years ago. This is love. This is sacrifice. This is compassion. This is life. This is what's called doing the right thing. Helping people like Lisa and her family is my passion and my mission with Leeza's Place.

When I first met Lisa, my initial thought was, damn, this girl has as much energy as I do. She possesses the passion and drive for the same cause: our fight against Alzheimer's disease. And to top it off, she's worked in television and is a multi-award winning author. She's also one of the youngest caregivers I've met, and I believe that is an invaluable commodity. What this disease needs are spokespeople with spunk...and Cerasoli lacks for none. But here's what else I realized: Lisa was not a person who had caregiving in her past, someone who had moved on to writing and public speaking. She's on the battlefront everyday. Her grandmother is eighty-nine and still with the family. Lisa is a pro in the care-giving arena. It just so happens that the worry, fear, utter exhaustion and hopelessness that most caregivers experience are not a part of her character. She and her family choose humor as their weapon of survival. And it shows on every page of her offbeat, honest, hilarious and touching memoir.

Alzheimer's should not be minimized as merely part of The Gray Wave that is crashing to shore. It's a tsunami of pain that is hushed up by those who find it taboo and dismissed by those who believe it's merely a part of getting older. I think those who are forgetting should not be forgotten, and we can't let fear immobilize us. In just over a decade, the number of people age sixty-five and older is going to double from 45 to 90 million. And that's just in the United States. Every 71 seconds another family gets the diagnosis, and death in slow motion begins. Caregivers are the ones who are leading the army of change while struggling to keep it all together. Because the "compassion fatigue" from which they suffer is so great, we are committed to helping them become educated, empowered and energized for their caregiving journey. That's what Leeza's Place is about.

I know from personal experience with my beautiful mother, Gloria Jean--and discuss it extensively in my book, Take Your Oxygen First--that the diagnosis of a dementia-related illness is shocking and heartbreaking news. It's a gut punch for which you can never be ready. And there is no happy ending. Not yet

I dare to say that Alzheimer's disease may have found its Tuesdays with Morrie in the memoir, As Nora Jo Fades Away. And with it comes our latest, greatest, witty, outspoken warrior against this illness: Lisa Cerasoli. She was "Called to Action." And she's stepped up to the task just like a real warrior--with her face paint on.

Give the girl a sword. She's got enemies to slay. And we can all laugh, cry, hope and believe with her 'til she gets the job done.

Prologue

So how was your day? I want a divorce. Looks like it might rain. Hey, check it out. I think my socks don't match.

It could have been anything. I was only half-listening.

"Stop the car."

"What?"

"Stop the car. I want out," I restated with an indifference odd even for me.

"Um, stopping sort of in the middle of nowhere would be weird. Hey, check it out, it's starting to drizzle … and my socks don't match!"

Yeah, that is weird.

The rain had begun to both pitter and patter delicately on the windshield. It felt like an imaginary imp had crawled inside my brain and was beating on my eardrum.

"And quit sounding nuts. You're killing a perfectly good joyride."

My body was as still as a marble chess piece. Then abruptly one arm swung fluidly over to the seatbelt latch, startling me back to life. The sound of the belt unbuckling clicked in perfect sync with either a pitter or a patter. Either way, it went unnoticed by that other "dude" robbing my alone space.

Meanwhile, a thumb drummed on the steering wheel in lazy rhythm with the song on the radio—Guns 'N Roses' "I Used to Love Her." This tune added stunning irony to my ongoing "pity party" and it seemed to drag on forever as if under direct order from the Universe to embed itself—word for word—into my gray matter.

I used to love her, oh yeah, but I had to kill her.
I used to love her, oh yeah, but I had to kill her.
I had to put her six feet under.
She's buried right in my backyard.
Ugh.

Then it occurred to me. I could steal those lyrics for this eulogy that's been mulling around my brain. I nearly laughed out loud at the thought of it—of burying "her" in the back yard (*and still hearing her complain*). But then I shivered and ultimately cringed. *Shit, am I going to Hell for thinking this?* Wouldn't be the first time that thought had crossed my mind either.

I peeked behind me. No traffic. What if I just slid out the door at seventy miles per hour? Bones would shatter, blood spew. Any idiot knows that, idiot!

A grave familiar numbness embodied me, wound around every inch of flesh like I had been mummified. *Breathe. Now cut the drama and nonsensical dialogue. It's after dark. You've made it through this day. Turn the car around.*

I flipped a bitch and headed home.

That's what it felt like living with dementia—like being trapped in a car heading nowhere while the same peculiar track plays over and over taunting, torturing, and tempting me to jump. All the while Reason bats at Emotion instigating a chronic wrestling match inside my head.

I was both driver and passenger in this new life I'd incited.

I mean, it was my "big idea" to move Grandma in. Yet it swiftly became apparent that my main job was to merely observe and occasionally alert that *other* guy (the driver—the one with the "big idea") of grave danger.

So with a lethal mix of hope and anxiety, I anticipated being struck silly by the notion that I am finally in OVER MY HEAD. But I'm not there yet. The water may be ear deep, but I'm sipping air with neck a'stretched.

One day Gram will wake in Heaven or wander into that new place where I'm no longer needed or known. Then at least the decisions that plague me daily would narrow themselves down with indisputable clarity.

But that day's not today. So I drive home and do what I've been doing. I wait.

As Nora Jo
Fades Away

Chapter One

"There's only one man I've ever loved.
We met when I was fourteen and we were married for sixty-seven years.
What the hell was his name?"

Nora Jo
March 31, 2008

Hospital Green
and the
Ben Gay Wing

*T*HE FIRST TWO MONTHS WERE THE hardest on me physically. I mostly brought it on myself. I mean, there was a "fall" that occurred a week into moving Grandma in, and that was terrifying. But other than that, the anxiety that infested my body was all mine to own.

As rapidly as a teenage girl forms her first real crush, moving Grandma in caused "Sleep" to become my premiere enemy. We weren't that close to begin with (Sleep and I), but having an on-again/off-again adversary blow in and out of my life was manageable. Having "It" move in permanently created a brand new world of the bizarre.

They say after three days of not sleeping a person can start hallucinating. This chronic deprivation can damage relationships, one's ability to concentrate, create short-term memory loss, irritability, and headaches. Driving can become a dangerous activity and drinking may qualify as a favored pastime for someone suffering from sleep deprivation. I have embraced all symptoms minus the hallucinating (I think) throughout the course of "Life with Gram."

April, 2008

THUD!

My husband and I gave each other a quick look of panic and madly raced from living room to kitchen. Gram lay on the floor—stiff, white and motionless. Our daughter was on top of her. We grabbed our scared, naked, speechless toddler and proceeded to utter Gram's name over and over.

"Nora? Nor? Can you hear me?" My very calm, cool, and collected husband inquired.

I was flipping out and chattering like a freak on the phone with a family member at the time (who was also flipping out and chattering all freak-like). "Gram, *Gram?* Are you okay? What happened? Do you need me to call an ambulance? Are you in pain? Can you breathe? Open your eyes? *Gram??*"

"Lisa, what the hell just happened? Is she okay? Do you need to call an ambulance? Is she opening her eyes? What's going on?!" the voice in the phone shouted back.

"Get off the phone." Mr. Rational suggested strongly.

A good suggestion, "I'll call you back."

"*Call me back!*"

Click.

"Honey, what happened?" Mr. Rational turned his attention to the kid.

"I was on the counter 'cause I wanted to make a ba-ba, easy-on-the-chocolate-warm-and-yummy, cause I'm a big girl and G.G. tried to pick me up and she went boom. Boom! I did not push her. She just went Boom! *G.G. are you okay ??*" Jazzlyn Jo yelled right into G.G.'s ear like she was deaf and/or dead. (G.G.: abbreviation for Great Grandma. I used it once in front of Jazz and it stuck like glue.)

"Shit, Gram. Shit." We've been telling her for months NOT to pick up the baby. I hadn't seen her do it since Christmas. I thought we didn't have to worry about this anymore. "How many beers do you think she's had, honey?"

"Well, it's only six o'clock, two, maybe three. Not enough to cushion the fall, just enough to make her believe she could do something stupid like pick up the kid," my husband Pete reasoned again.

"Gram, do you want to go to the hospital?" I asked slowly and audibly, mimicking Jazz.

"No, no." She opened her eyes, touched her heart. God, she was pale. "Just let me lay here and catch my breath."

"What were you thinking? You know you can't pick up the baby!" Okay, she's alive. I'm free to scream and scold. But then relief overcame me and I quickly mellowed. "Listen, I'll grab a pillow for your head and your legs. Do you hurt anywhere?"

"My back, my back."

"Don't worry, Nor. We've got you. You lie right here. We'll

get you comfortable until you're ready to move. Want me to grab your beer? You could drink it through a straw till you feel recovered enough to get up."

She smiled up at Pete. He has always had a way with her. It was momentarily reassuring. Then she nodded "yes" to his question—which was slightly less comforting.

She laid there for another hour, catching her breath and yes … *sipping her beer*. Finally, Pete moved her to the couch until bedtime (which for Gram was midnight or a six pack later, whichever came first).

We ended up at the ER the next morning. There were three hairline fractures in her L4. Of course, with advanced osteoporosis and without a recent X-ray, it was impossible to determine if the fractures were a result of this specific accident.

It was a six–week recovery. We served up mounds and mounds *and mounds* of Darvocets on demand. The first three weeks entailed a lot of lifting on my part—to and from the bed and the toilet, sometimes in the middle of the night. One night, I didn't hear her moan, groan, or whatever you want to call it, and she didn't want to yell, so she pissed in my favorite coffee mug (which I had lovingly left by her bedside with a touch of drinking water).

We definitely felt like we had created a real calamity. She had been so able-bodied before the move. Now, just two short weeks later, I'm lifting her up and putting on her socks and underwear and helping her maneuver everywhere. Meanwhile she's gulping down Darveys (everything gets a nickname in this joint) like my kid pops Tic-Tacs and pissing in my favorite coffee mug. And, as far as we could tell, she was kosher with all of this. Maybe the Darveys had her in a mood (as in an *I-don't-give-a-shit mood*).

Good-bye, favorite coffee mug, I thought that morning as I backed out of the garage to head into work. Pete chased me up the driveway, waving it wildly. "Honey, honey, I just washed it! You want me to fill it up for ya?" He was laughing his ass off, and after three scary weeks, finally so was I.

Helping Gram physically was a piece of cake. I mean, she weighed "a buck twenty-five." But there were a series of other things that put a constant strain on both my conscience and soul. Like:

1. Living with the fear she might never recover.

2. Feeling responsible for her fall.

3. Wishing I had moved her in one week earlier or later and changed fate.

4. Wondering if I was incapable of looking after her. And...

5. Thinking that at any given moment the woman might croak. I mean, she has reached croaking age.

As a result of my brain working in constant overdrive, I didn't sleep for two solid months. Every single night in bed I lay with eyes wide open, listening like a guard on graveyard shift at the state penitentiary waiting for a prison break. I took my job *that* seriously. There'd be a snore. *Is she choking?* A wheeze. *Did she stop breathing?* A creek. *Crap, is she trying to get up? Is she going to fall again? And who's going to stop talking to me NEXT over all this rigmarole?*

You can't move her in. Are you crazy? Are you looking to get divorced? That's what they invented nursing homes for. You are not a nurse. She is not your responsibility. She's not even your mother, just your grandmother. No one will blame you for putting her in a home. But don't move her in. We tried it. You CANNOT do it. It will ruin your marriage. Or, at the very least, you WILL go nuts. Trust us, we know So-n-So, they tried it and THEY WENT NUTS ... and got divorced.

Opinions flew freely from every direction. And they danced inside my head late night and sardonically.

My mother Sherie had volunteered over and over to move in permanently with Gram. She meant it, too. She sincerely did. She had been sleeping there several nights a week for the last two years anyway. She was amazing. But the sleepovers mostly entailed her rolling in after dinner with friends, putting up with an hour of senseless irrational chatter and CNN at a decibel level I think they use for torture in some countries, and then escaping early morning before the senseless, endless irrational chatter began all over again. She also cleaned her house and paid all her bills, too. Again—*amazing*. But there was a limit to the "down time" she could handle with her mom-in-law.

The problem was that she and Gram could not maintain ongoing pleasantries for more than a couple of minutes since the death of my dad (my mother's husband, my grandmother's youngest son). There was too much pain between them. They looked at each other and all they saw was "Dickie." All they felt was the presence of a guy that was no longer in the room tugging ruthlessly at their hearts, leaving the air between them thick and at war over "*who missed him more.*"

They shared a mutual and justifiable adoration for the guy when he was alive (I'm talking about that crazy unconditional love that you read about in really great literature). Then he was tragically removed from their lives. Yet somehow whenever these two women got together, Dickie would creep right into the room and then linger with an edgy influence. Certainly that must qualify as some form of torture. I can tell you it's been hard to witness, even with my eyes closed while CNN assaults my auditory faculties.

I couldn't do that to my two favorite women. I could not allow these angelic creatures who raised me to be trapped together forever losing a never-ending wrestling match to a dead guy, and then watch them take that defeat out on each other. I could not allow these generous, modest, loving women to have "grief" be the inescapable theme of their lives. And I was pretty certain living under the same roof would ensure that. There's enough pain, lethargy, insecurity and anger that comes with that heavy-duty emotion under normal circumstances. If an environment were created that thrived parasite-like because of it, a deep, irreversible hostility both passive and aggressive would inevitably become the ultimate derailment of both their existences.

So what do you know? It was up to me after all.

She kept odd hours, Nora Josephine Cerasoli, my eighty-seven year old grandmother. That too messed royally with my shut-eye. Slowly though, the initial unusualness of it became common and even quite workable for our lifestyle. It's ended up being a small perk buried beneath the enormous stifling change.

But during those first two months, before I felt comfortable with her schedule and became somewhat "cool" in the knowledge that the odd hours were in fact a product of her disease and depression, pure and simple, I was indeed a frazzled insomniac, a maniacal mess. I was the chick with the mirror searching for breath if she didn't rise up to meet the world by 10:30 in the morning. Jazz, my vivacious and precocious near-three-year-old joined me in my musings. Sneaking into someone's bedroom while they're sleeping to hold a mirror over their face to see if they're still breathing was our grand new morning adventure. And Jazz was thrilled. *Blues Clues* had nothin' on this event.

"Mommy, is it time yet? I'll get the mirror!" She'd dash into the bathroom, her adorable, animated, bare-butted self. Then she'd beeline, mirror in hand, for G.G.'s room.

I'd race to catch up. "Quiet, Jazz. Quiet. Be very quiet, lovey."

Jazz would attempt to hold it steady. I usually took over, not wanting G.G. to get spucked in the face with a big ol' mirror. Can you imagine waking up from a deep slumber to your own face staring back you from an inch away? Eighty-seven or not, that'd be seriously freaky.

"Is she alive?" She'd whisper all wide-eyed, not seeming to actually care which way it went. I mean, the reality of the outcome was lost on her. What can you expect?

"Yes, Jazz, she's alive. See the mirror? It's fogging up from her breath. Now let's go."

We'd tiptoe out.

Okay, so Gram didn't die today. Now go live your life, do some yoga, clean your house, read to the kid, walk the freaking dog. Write—there's a thought. Sleep—an even more brilliant idea.

But I couldn't sleep.

Moving in with "The Weavers" really went down like more of a rescue mission. She had spent most weekends for the last two years being lugged up to the house anyway. The place was utterly familiar to her. And the surroundings were comfortable, especially for maneuvering around.

One day, about a week prior to the long-debated move/rescue mission, she confessed that she had almost set her house on fire. Apparently, she left chicken thighs cooking for like a day-and-a-half at four hundred and fifty degrees. Then she broke into a string of irrational ruminations as she sat at her kitchen table tugging and twisting each hand like she was extracting water from them.

"The Iraqis have poisoned my lettuce. I had to throw it away. *See?*" She got up and shoved her hand into the garbage and pulled out half a head of lettuce. And there it was—proof that the Iraqis did in fact poison it. Then she went on to confide that they (the Iraqis) had sneaked in the night before and stolen a drawer full of kitchen towels. Naturally, she then opened the drawer that normally housed the kitchen towels and, sure enough, it was empty. Then she fled back to the bathroom and came out with a jar full of tweezers (somewhere in the neighborhood of twenty).

"Can you tell me what these are? They're just sitting in my bathroom. What am I supposed to be doing with them?" she questioned with panicked sincerity.

You should know that I had already personally witnessed "the plucking of the chin hair" for what seemed like my entire existence. The tweezers were at the pinnacle of the decision to move her in.

She also spoke frankly and evenly about the walls closing in—moving right at her. She said she could see them doing it *now*, and asked if I'd also noticed them "making their move." I told her I did not. But I understood what she meant. And, frankly, that part didn't seem all that crazy to me, mostly just sad. The "tweezers" and "Iraqis" though? They were cause for pause.

Assisted living was simply out of the question. Gram is many things: generous, hard-working, extremely welcoming, but stubborn and controlling rank up there, too (just below paranoid). Moving in with us was within her realm of reality and well inside her safety zone. We promised to move her favorite bedroom furniture and arrange it like it was in her old place, and within twenty-four hours of her strange admissions, the "rescue mission" was complete.

We also asked her to pick out paint for her new room. Bedroom-wise, it was either Jazz or Brock (Pete's teenage son) who'd have to be minus a bedroom until we finished the downstairs, so Jazz obviously lost that coin toss. We had no real options. She moved into the master bedroom … and was thrilled!

Us? Not so much.

Anyway, we didn't want to have Gram living between princess-pink walls, so we needed to repaint. She picked a color called Rejuvenation. It was this summery, soothing green. I was so excited. Of course, by the time we got all her "stuff" in there—the old-time photos, the porcelain figurine of an old couple swinging on a bench (it plays "Memories" when you wind it—which Jazz does frequently), a glass statue of the Virgin Mary, several rosaries to grace the dresser tops along with as many Kleenex boxes and a Bible so huge it could kill a small dog if directly dropped on top of it— "Rejuvenation" quickly took on a color I begrudgingly began referring to as Hospital Green.

So Gram got her cozy room in the lovely shade of "hospital green" at the end of our ranch-style home which was soon designated by my husband as "The Ben Gay Wing."

How long is she staying? Over and over we got that question. I finally started answering, "A year. She's staying a year. Anyone can do anything for a year, right?" And people had a tendency to be satisfied with that response.

I still wasn't sleeping though. At all.

June 5, 2008

I sat on the crunchy white paper on the cool hard examining table, all hunched over with my elbows on my knees, chin cupped in hands, ready to beg for a sedative and pull out the water works if need be.

All I wanted was immediate reprieve. Couldn't think beyond that. *Just give me one Valium (like the size of a gumdrop) to knock me out long enough so that functioning semi-coherently could be part of my existence again—if only for a day.*

No begging necessary. Doc took one look at me and set me up with this lovely Paxil-Klonopin cocktail. It saved my life, my marriage, my sanity (well, sort of) and the physical well-being of all parties cohabitating under the Weaver roof, at least for the summer. I was a new woman, a rested woman, and I was able to manage Gram and her little peculiarities and peccadilloes with an ease and patience I didn't know existed inside the "walls of Lisa."

And life weirdly forged on, but not so much forward as sideways.

Chapter Two

"We Plan, God Laughs."

Sherre Hirsch
Best-selling Author
*We Plan, God Laughs: Ten Steps to Finding Your Divine Path
When Life is not Turning out like You Wanted*

Captured and Caged

PRIOR TO MOVING BACK TO MY hometown of Iron Mountain, Michigan, I pretty much led a life of self-servitude.

Our thirteenth amendment guarantees freedom from involuntary servitude. Servitude means to be enslaved, and my personal interpretation of self-servitude as applied to the life I lived pre-Michigan was that I was *enslaved* to myself. I was a full-time prisoner to my very own hopes, dreams, and ambitions. I was single, living in Los Angeles, and pursuing an acting and writing career full throttle. I had a whole heap of worries, don't get me wrong. But they were all related to me: Lisa, single chick, career-minded woman, dream catcher.

When I took that unexpected turn in the fall of 2002 on the highway headed to nowhere and landed in Michigan to care for my ailing father, I did not expect to stay. I expected to "heal" the guy (silly little human that I am), and go back to life as usual.

But *Someone* had other plans for me.

July 24, 2003

"Who is this guy?" My grandfather asked as he gazed at my father's obituary in *The Daily News*.

"He was a friend of yours." I exhaled the lie proficiently into a room crammed with relatives, a room that had been abruptly and agonizingly silenced by his innocent inquiry.

"Yeah, yeah. I think I liked that guy," he said nodding.

"We all liked him, Gramps," I choked out, then patted his back as he casually shifted to the sports section.

My mother and I, along with the rest of the family, worked in shifts to help Gram with Gramps immediately following my father's death. But Gramps was on a rapid decline and it was tough. In less than a year, Alzheimer's claimed his life. His sweet soul was finally free to join his son's in the tranquil blue Heavens. And for that I was grateful. My dad was no longer all alone up there.

So, within eleven months of my father's death on July 20, 2003, we buried my grandfather. In the meantime, I had become a wife and stepmom (and was soon-to-be pregnant). And between all that, Pete's dad fell victim to lung cancer as well. The disease specifically claimed Jack Weaver's life six days before our September wedding. My former life turned into an elusive hallucination. And this new one could be most accurately described in Hollywood terms as a certifiable MOW (Movie of the Week).

Acting was no longer an option, so I continued to write (when

I found the time for it) and loved that. But I went from happily renting a room in a friend's condo to maintaining a four-bedroom house complete with a yard. *A yard*?

I had forgotten the work owning a house complete with a f$@#&%g yard entailed and was clueless about the true time-suck having a family meant. I still to this day don't know how any woman gives birth to more than one child. Who has the time? So my life of self-servitude lost its prefix quicker than I could blink an eye. I was now down to just "servitude."

I was a hamster racing fervently on the wheel-runner of life—sort of like the rest of the world—except I didn't want to be like the rest of the world. Yet there I was consumed by my new career as a professional juggler. I juggled baby, bills, house, work, housework, hubby, a grieving mother and grandmother, and tried somewhere between it all to fit in time for that girl I used to know—Lisa the career-minded woman, dream catcher.

Mostly, my life was too jammed with "busy work" to perform any activity with the proficiency I knew myself to be capable of in that *other* life, never mind trying to squeeze in "the dream." But I did manage occasionally to sneak back into the world I so missed by catching a good movie, working on a script, or chatting with a friend out west.

When that didn't happen (which was a lot), I felt somewhat "stuck" inside this life that was foreign and didn't quite fit right, like when you play dress up in Mom's closet. It's magical until you get hungry, tired, bored, lonely, or disappointed in the limited options and same old accessories. Then you realize that even after another proud year of growth, the clothes still don't look right. They weren't meant for you, why should they? Except now (welcome to adulthood) you can't strip them off and be free. But I *did* manage. I juggled and maintained … until Grandma moved in.

And that's the thing about juggling. There's a limit to how many balls you can keep dancing in the air. So maybe it wasn't Nora Jo specifically. Maybe it was that I could not handle having one more thing to do.

Moving her in solidified the notion that I was officially tethered to this new life that hadn't been tailored for me yet. So, in addition to severe and certain insomnia and anxiety that had me rubbing my heart as routinely as bathroom breaks, I was beginning to feel resentful and regretful … and genuinely caged.

The Summer of 2008

I quickly discovered to my surprise and chagrin that the only thing harder than taking care of someone who doesn't want to die is taking care of someone who does.

Since the death of her husband and son, Nora Jo has wanted nothing more than to be done with this earthly existence. And as sure as an alarm clock wakes you for the workday, she'd beg God or one of us to please help her get out of here (planet Earth). Unfortunately for my gram, her date with demise was yet to be set. She didn't have cancer. Nothing tangibly terminal. I could not assure her of an efficient six-month exit date. In fact, I couldn't guarantee her much of anything. I'd just tell her God has a plan for all of us and He must want Jazzy to know her great grandmother,

her "G.G." That was the best rationale I could scrounge up.

That last theory has become so overused even the woman who can't remember her husband's name has grown sick of hearing it.

I remember quite vividly my father crying daily, consumed by the timbre of death's dark horse galloping ever more near. My grandmother now cried for lack of it. This quickly explained the excessive sleeping. She wandered our house aimlessly and awkwardly as if she hadn't spent every single weekend for the better part of two years here.

She immediately lost interest in cooking, her one and only pastime. My husband could get her hooked on peeling a potato or two when he worked his way about the kitchen, but she initiated nothing.

I forced her to continue to make her own coffee every morning. At first, she was *not* happy about waking up and *not* having it pre-brewed (when clearly the rest of us were bustling around well into our day). And I found that strange for several reasons:

1. She's always been a real worker, you know, a child-of-the-depression workaholic.

2. She lived alone for four years after my Grandpa Fritz passed away. That's over a thousand days worth of brewing coffee. And …

3. She spent sixty-seven years prior to that making him coffee. In fact, one of her favorite sayings regarding Grandpa Fritz has always been, *Poor guy couldn't even make himself a cup a' coffee. 'Course it's not his fault. I never took the time to teach him.*

But somehow this notion that people were up and about and

17

didn't have coffee ready-made struck a sour chord with her.

It was important to me, however, no matter how depressed she grew, that she maintain "the skills of living" which included dressing herself, making coffee, reading, gardening, and maintaining mobility (*e.g.*, walking and getting in and out of chairs).

The elderly have a tendency to lose upper body strength. It is the number one reason why "they fall and can't get up." I did not want that happening to Gram. I admit it looked like cruel and unusual punishment when someone watched her try (a half dozen times) to get out of her special rocker/recliner while I sat on the sidelines silently rooting her on, offering no assistance. But I wasn't about to budge on the importance of mobility. Not yet.

In fact, I sometimes feel as if a lot of our daily rituals seem unusual and even cruel. But trying to get someone to remain "sane" just a little bit longer—when time and disease are performing the opposite task disturbingly more effectively—is a constant battle. And trying to get that same person (the one who wishes every minute of every day she were dead) to read a magazine, go for a walk, take a ride to the market, watch a movie, take a bath or simply get out of bed, is exhausting. It's like training for a marathon you know you'll never get to run. The phrase, *I don't know why someone doesn't just take me out back and shoot me?* has been uttered more in the past year than "good morning," "good night," and "get me a beer." After a while, it becomes just one more thing that's carried out the door with my day:

Grab purse, keys, lunch, and hope Gram is alive when I return, or hope maybe she's dead ... because she wants to be ... I think?

Am I going to go to Hell for thinking this? Oh, shut up.

I don't know what I think.

I do know that living with someone this depressed makes me feel like I'm carrying around five extra pounds after Christmas that I just can't shake. It's all in my gut and it affects the way I walk, my general self image, and even lowers the desire to squeeze into my favorite figure-friendly jeans. It has, in fact, lowered my desire for just about everything (except the drive not to end up like her—the woman whom I've worshipped my entire life).

I can see from her demeanor—the hard and heavy energy that has encapsulated her—that she's carrying a bit more than just Christmas weight. She may never have had a driver's license, but one thing is for certain, Nora Jo was the star of her own show when she had the gumption and the right audience. She was also the leader of a tightly knit pack (her family) before death struck two of its hugely significant members.

And she cooked. As president of the clan, that was her noteworthy contribution. The woman owned two kitchens. She made a full-time job out of selling Italian food and pasties (pies stuffed with meat, potatoes, and veggies—a handheld meal created for miners). Then in her spare time, she squeezed in three meals a day for the family. She never tired, never complained, and she never ran out of food.

I can't recall with even slight accuracy how many times I've watched her whip out two dozen pasties or twelve dozen raviolis without breaking a sweat or smudging her perfectly applied L'Oreal lipstick in the vivacious shade of Satin Berry. And I never saw her without a smile on her face (not until the day my dad died).

She had one of those faces that welcomed you into her home and convinced you to stay for dinner all with one grin. She was that good, that bighearted.

That was then.

Now I had taken away her kitchen. I had taken away *both* kitchens. I mean, it wasn't me, but to someone who's losing their mind, it might seem that way. And she was drained, confused, and the saddest woman to still be breathing. "Free time" overwhelmed her. It was her enemy. In her new surroundings—the one minus her two personalized kitchens—she was now given all the time in the world to exercise the art of perfecting her role as "saddest woman alive." When she felt like talking, which was always, she'd bitch or cry about the loss of everything. At least she still had the tact to accuse "them" and "they" rather than "me" and "mine" when she went off on a rant:

"I think they rented my house."

"They won't go pick up my favorite swing."

"They ran out of bread. I sure hope they get some for tomorrow. I can't eat my eggs without bread."

"I love that bush with the pink flowers in my yard. Why won't they go dig it up?"

"They wouldn't let me drink last night. They said I had a cough. What's a beer gonna do to hurt a cough? They're nuts."

"You know they sold my house ... just sold it! Now I'll never get that pink bush."

Any day, August, 2008

"How come *they* didn't make any coffee?" Nora Jo grumbled, mostly to herself.

"You know how to make it, Gram." I exhaled evenly.

"This isn't my house. I don't know where you keep your damned coffee."

"Sure you do. I put everything in the cupboard above the coffee maker, above your coffee maker. You know how to do it. You've been doing it for five months now," I'd add, not making eye contact, masking frustration.

"It's one o'clock. Somebody should have made some damned coffee by now." In a flash, she'd change her tone and life would be back to normal. Well, by normal I mean a bizarre cross between a Norman Rockwell painting and some random episode of *All in the Family.*

"It's one o'clock? Shit, half the day's gone," she'd chuckle. "It's almost time for a drink."

"You working it out over there, Gram?"

"I'll figure it out, dear. Your old Grandma still has a couple of marbles knocking together up here," she'd add, tapping her head.

"You know we don't drink coffee, Gram. Well, Pete doesn't and I'm a decaf girl."

"A what? Who the hell doesn't drink coffee? Never heard of such a thing."

Then she'd mull around, start making coffee, and mumble, "To each his own." This phrase has become the glue that fills the gap between our respective generations like moss on a rock trapped indefinitely between land and pond.

By four o'clock in the afternoon, we were generally in the clear for a few hours. She was settled into her recliner with a mug full of brandy & water as CNN blared throughout our living area.

She had moved in with all the basic old lady essentials ... plus two cases of brandy. And let me tell ya, *Bartley's* kept us busy all summer.

There was no stopping the drinking. We gave up that fight pretty early on. But we did try to get clever.

Mr. Peter Weaver and I always made sure to hold on to the last empty fifth so that we could drain half of the new one into it and dilute the both of them with water. She never caught onto the game, just upped the amount of glasses she'd consume. It felt like a constant race. On the nights we lost, one of us was bound to find her rolling around her bedroom floor naked from the ankles up.

You know how most people usually fall asleep in their clothes when they drink too much? Well Gram was trapped by ritual. She needed those flannel pajamas no matter how drunk, except that the brandy/dementia combo frequently had her forgetting to take off her shoes *before* she pulled down her pants/long underwear/my grandfather's Fruit of the Loom BVDs she proudly and religiously converted to wearing since the day he died.

Mostly, I was the one who caught her naked. Mostly. But it was on those off nights when I'd hear the roar, "Your gram's rolling around her room naked again! You might want to go do something about that!" I felt bad for my husband, Saint Peter.

Speaking of saint-like entities, our friends have been beyond stellar, little angels floating in and out of our certifiably crazy abode bringing open arms, genuine smiles, and massive amounts of liquor. And they always came solidly geared up for the same old circular conversations with Gram, as if it were all brand new to them.

Without fail, that conversation entailed an initial introduction, a lengthy *do-you-remember-me* exchange of pleasantries that got really silly after the twentieth or thirtieth time, but nonetheless was the precursor to ALL succeeding communications. This was trailed by never-ending commentary from Gram explaining (with painful elaboration) who exactly she was and why she was living with us. Then, all that babble was wrapped neatly up with a lengthy synopsis of her entire life.

"Oh, sure, I think I remember you. I'm the Grandma. I used to live in town by the police department, but the kids, God bless 'em, they moved me up here when I could no longer live on my own. I'm over ninety years old, you know."

"Really, Nor? Are you that old? You're looking good, lady," one of Pete's buddies would say with a smirk.

"Oh, yes. Well, thank you." She gobbled that compliment up every time, but would then grow immediately forlorn. "You know I'm all alone. I lost my husband to that goddamned cancer when he was just young ..."

"He was eighty-seven, Gram. He died in his sleep. He didn't have cancer." I'd interject without making eye contact.

"To each his own," she'd say, brushing me off with a wave of her hand. "Well, he died, and I'm all alone. You know I met him when I was fourteen. Only man I ever kissed."

"I know, Nor, you said that last time I was here. *Yesterday.*"

"Yes. We met at the roller rink. He was such a good dancer. He was an instructor there, you know. Best dancer in town. We met when I was just fourteen. Only man I ever kissed ..."

"*Only man I ever kissed.*" I'd imitate.

We'd all chuckle and exchange looks as Nora Jo's monologue would inevitably trail into more of an introspective soliloquy, serving as her second most common form of self comfort. It was sweet, even the fortieth time around. She was in a state of bliss when she reminisced.

But, upon realizing most of us were still there and within earshot but no longer "listening" to her ramblings, she'd turn and crack open her latest primary soother—a warm Busch Light.

These evenings generally ended and/or erupted in song—one song specifically. This song has embedded itself even into the brain of my Jazzy. "Let's Make Believe That We're Happy" by Kitty Wells.

It's a country tune. Two lovers are having an affair behind both their significant others' backs. They love neither the ones they're with nor each other. But they will stop at nothing to make believe that their love is real for as long as they have to ... *until they make it come true.*

It's quite the song for someone who's "only ever kissed one man and been in love with him since she was fourteen." But that was her song. And it was guaranteed that if you were bold enough to brave Chez Weaver after six o'clock in the evening, you were assured a dose or two or three of Kitty Wells.

And that was summer.

The weather helped much more than I realized at the time.

Chapter Three

*"No beer cans or silverware
in the microwave.
Thanks."*

Lisa
September, 2008

The Lap Dog Theory

September, 2008

SIX MONTHS. WE'VE MADE IT SIX MONTHS and with very few battle wounds to show for it. Well, the microwave had a couple, but we humans were scar-free, visually anyway. And Gram was maneuvering around pretty much the way she did before the kitchen incident.

Her switch from brandy and water to Busch Light was a huge relief. Anyone who has ever been drunk knows it's a lot more challenging to get obliterated drinking light beer compared to hard alcohol. We were relieved for the conversion. The fact that she demanded the beer be "warm" was another story. September ultimately became known as "Microwave Awareness Month." Again, we found ourselves working in shifts.

I personally yanked half a dozen cans of Busch Light out of that contraption in four weeks' time. My mother stopped her on as many occasions as well. All the explaining in the world did

NOTHING ... well nothing but piss her off. By month's end, our new microwave boasted several impressive wall-to-wall singe marks. But worse than that was the worry of what happens after a "singe mark?" Would that be fire? An explosion? Would the gadget literally fly into pieces like shrapnel from a bomb and embed itself into anything within its path? Was I going to come home one day to my new gram? *Gram without a face?*

Yikes.

Finally, I thought about it. The woman can read, so I'll write a note. And I did. That note was in dark print on a bright orange Post-it:

NO BEER CANS OR SILVERWARE
IN THE MICROWAVE
THANKS

Then I affixed it permanently to the front of the microwave right next to the latch. It became quickly apparent that unless you were blind, it was impossible to open the microwave without reading the note. To everyone's relief, it cured the obsession she had with nuking cans of beer. It also hasn't seemed to bother or embarrass her. And this note has made for fabulous commentary amongst guests. So that problem was solved. Yay me.

Next ...

Gram hated being alone.

A social worker warned us before the rescue mission that she'd need her "space." He said we needed to make sure that there was a TV and a comfortable rocker in her bedroom. That way, she'd have a place of refuge. Allegedly, those were the two state requirements when taking on the task of housing and caring for an elderly person: they have to have a rocker and a TV. We (Mom and I) assured him that we'd oblige (rule abiders that we are), but that in Gram's case, it would NOT be necessary.

There, in Gram's room sits a comfortable rocker hidden under bundles of old sweaters that are filed under neither the "clean" nor the "dirty" category. I am not to touch them. And in near proximity of that is a TV that I've heard turned on once. *Hannah Montana* blared from it while Jazz jumped on the bed and Gram dug through her drawers looking for jewelry, her hearing aids, candy bars, or some other weird shit she'd either squirreled away or just plain lost.

There has never been any such thing as her "space." And damn if we weren't on point about that. If she woke up and no one was home yet, we heard about it for the whole rest of that day.

One day, amongst all my generally futile searches, I read on the Internet that the elderly adored lap dogs. It gave them a source of companionship, something to love and look after. Often times, it increased their awareness and revived the sense of purpose that was previously buried along with their long-lost loved ones. This applied particularly and specifically to people suffering from various forms of dementia including Alzheimer's.

Okay, so here's hoping the Internet knows my gram better than the social worker because at this stage in the game, I was willing to try anything for a little relief.

And so we got that lap dog and named him "Beau." He was an eight-week-old Tea Cup Poodle, a big-time snuggler, and true to his reputation, he wanted nothing more out of life than to curl up on someone's lap.

She had no use for him.

The rat. That thing. Those were a few of his nicknames. She'd also frequently refer to him as "Brock" (Pete's son and the other living being she wasn't particularly endeared to under our roof).

In her mind, that one-and-a-half pound ball of black fur was no more family than, well, Brock. What would the point of projecting love and energy toward either one of them prove? It would prove to be a waste of love and energy. That was her logic. And she also felt that both of these non-blood entities distracted from the constant fixation she had with Jazz. Fortunately, both Brock and Beau were generally ignored by Nora Jo, unless they tried to eat, that is. *And that's a whole 'nother story.*

But here we were thinking that a small dog would engage her senses, win her heart, and give her the one thing everybody desires—a sense of purpose.

She used to own a dog—a golden retriever like our other dog, Lucky. Apparently Gram loved her so much it was rumored the dog ate "three squares a day." Whatever meal Gram was cooking, the dog was eating right alongside her and my grandfather. Based on the platefuls of food we've caught her feeding Lucky, I think there might be some truth in that tale.

But her "purpose" in regard to Beau was to lock him in our bedroom. That was when she was in a good mood. If her mood wasn't so pleasant, like when she woke up hungover, she'd bat at him with a foot and snarl things like, *What do you want? I got nothing for you. Why don't you go outside? Maybe a bear will have you for breakfast and we'll be done with you.* ... And so on.

Gram's no longer allowed to put the dog outside (there are actually bear out there). And Beau figured out all on his own it'd be best to hang out in our bedroom closet until someone returned with a "lap" that could be of use to him.

He's up to a little over three pounds now, that adorable little critter. The vet says he's full grown and perfectly healthy. The truth is Beau's a survivor, plain and simple, just like Brock. Just like the rest of us.

October 2008

My brother Rick, his wife Jen, and new baby Jakey visit often. They're from the Detroit area and he's been out of work for six months. While it's been a gigantic burden for him financially, as it has been for so many families across America, we felt (on a selfish note) so lucky and relieved to get to see them so much, particularly at this juncture in our existence.

It had been two months since their last visit, and Rick immediately noticed and fell in mad-love with the new addition of the orange Post-it. He spent hours prepping and planning his assault on the microwave. As soon as I'd walk into the kitchen— BAM—he'd pop a beer can into it. Then he'd read the sign aloud, look at me in utter dismay, and crack up. It was great.

What wasn't so great was that Gram didn't know who the hell Rick was. She called him every name under the sun for the first of his two-week stay: Leonard, Bart, Pete, Brock, Jeff, Justin, Dickie, That-Big-Fat-Guy-With-The-Tattoo.

My brother has a funky tattoo wrapped around his right bicep. And, yes, one could qualify him as "big." But he's big as in, *I'm a bad ass. Don't mess with me. He's not big like, Hey, I just won the annual hot dog eating contest down at the county fair.*

Nonetheless, if you weren't "rail thin," in Gram's eyes, YOU WERE FAT. There was no middle ground, no "healthy" looking people in her world, just she and I (the thin ones) and everyone else, the fatties. And she loved her similes. *He's huge as a horse. She's big as a house. Her ass is as wide as a car. He looks like he's about to give birth to twins. And her fave: She's got an ass out to here.* That's when she'd stretch her arms as far apart as they could possibly go.

Of course, as a relevant side note, her obsession with "slenderly-challenged" did not come as a result of dementia. She actually went through a phase when her ass was getting to be "out to here," too. And she'd joke about it ... but then go walk five miles. This disease has merely served as a catalyst to set a long-standing prejudice joyfully free. That among other social faux pas was an integral part of her colloquialisms. Basically, the woman never had a "thought" she kept to herself.

She had this old friend, Ilene. Ilene and Gram were the same exact age, although Ilene had experienced a bit more wear 'n tear over the years. There were four houses on Gram's entire block, three of which Gram had personally rented, owned, or lived in. Those homes were all white. Ilene's house was not. Between that and the fact that Ilene had lived there for over fifty years, we all knew Ilene. Yet every time Gram spoke of her, she used the same lengthy intro as if the rest of us wouldn't know who the hell the poor woman was without the added commentary:

"You know my friend Ilene? Teeth so yellow they're green? Yeah, she brought me flowers today. She sure is sweet. Tough old broad, too. And teeth so ..."

"Yeah, Gram, we get it. Ilene brought you flowers. They're beautiful."

In case you were wondering, as I was, why Gram had lived in three of the four houses on that block throughout her life, I asked her one day. She replied, "I liked the neighborhood. Why ruin a good thing?"

About two days prior to Rick's departure, I noticed Gram sitting in her favorite rocker crying silently over CNN and a coffee mug full of warm beer.

"Gram, you okay? What's wrong?"

"I'm just so ashamed."

"Of what, Gram? What happened?"

"That's Ricky. That big man in this house, that's our Ricky."

"I know Gram. That's your grandson, my brother."

"I know. I know." She blew her nose, then scratched at a tear with a Satin Berry nail. "I didn't realize till just this minute that he's my Ricky. I'm just so ashamed of myself."

"There's nothing to be ashamed of, Gram. It's not your fault. You have dementia. Remember? You're losing your memory, that's why you live with me. I'm your memory now, Gram. It's okay."

"It's not okay."

"Gram, it is okay. This happens to lots of people your age. Like fifty percent of people your age suffer from memory loss."

"Yeah, but eighty percent of 'em are already dead."

She had a point.

She continued to cry, too, inconsolably. My brother walked in, cold beer in hand. "Hey, Gram, what's up?"

I gave him a look, but waited for her version of the predicament.

"Ricky, oh Ricky, I just realized that you're my Ricky. I'm so ashamed. I'm so sorry."

"It's okay, Gram. I don't mind."

"But I mind. I wasted all this time wondering who this big man in my house was ... and it was you." And she was just crying all over the place. "You're my Ricky, Dickie's son. My grandson. I'm so ashamed."

"Hey, Gram, let's cut the crap. Cut the whining. I'm okay. You're okay. We're all here. You know who I am. Now why don't you get your ass out of that chair and join me in the kitchen for a beer. We can talk about the good ol' days and shit. C'mon now, Gram."

"Okay," she conceded, smiling, sniffling and nodding.

Rick took her gently by the arm and escorted her into the kitchen.

They spent the rest of the evening reminiscing about the neighborhood, the day she met Gramps (at fourteen), the birth of Dickie, and other long-overstated stories we all knew too well.

Her tears quickly dried on top of cheeks that remained

permanently hoisted by a bright unbroken smile as she fell deep and hard into the glorious vivid lucidity of her long gone past.

Rick listened as if it was all brand new.

Gram felt like "herself" for the rest of that night.

And I, too, was free to relax, although I was beginning to lose sight of what exactly that meant anymore. I cracked a Killian's, grabbed my latest form of escapism, *Eat, Pray, Love* by Elizabeth Gilbert, and pondered the notion while I curled up on the couch.

It wasn't long before Kitty Wells erupted as background music for yet another Night-In-The-Life. I smiled to myself relieved for a couple of reasons:

1. Gram was happy. And …

2. Thankfully, Gram could actually sing.

It was sweet. She could hold a steady little tune with the perfect amount of "twang" hooked onto the end of each and every verse. And away she went for round two.

Let's make believe that we're happy.

Let's pretend that I love you,

Let's make believe till we can make it come true.

You belong to another,

And I belong to someone, too.

I can't seem to feel, that my love for you is real,

Let's make believe till we can make it come true ...

*"This IS my first beer. It's my FIRST
beer after my LAST beer."*

Nora Jo
Four beers into any given Friday

The Little Gold Coin

ARCH 18, 1921. THAT WAS THE day the Lord graced John and Mary with their third baby girl. Nora Josephine McMahon was named directly after her grandmother on her father's side of the family and was eighth in a string of twelve children. Gram's fondness for singing dates pretty much back to birth. Her mother, Mary, was a self-taught guitarist and also played the harmonica or, in Gram's words, the mouth organ. As a product of the Depression, the family relied mainly on love and song to stay afloat. So between her mother's musical proclivities and the woman's "self-made" crowd, entertainment at the McMahon farm house was only a sunset away.

Nora never made it past junior high. She can't remember if her parents needed her to take care of her smaller siblings or if they simply didn't have enough clothes for all the girls to wear to school, but those were the two reasons that stood out. Either way, she didn't think twice about it.

Her first and only employer was Montgomery Ward, a department store she could easily walk to from her Iron Mountain home (you know, one of those three white houses). She maintained this job for nearly two decades, until a chair broke from under her during one of her shifts and permanently injured her lower back. After that, she received about forty dollars every two weeks in workman's compensation (a check that went religiously into a savings account for the next twenty years). It was at this point that she conceptualized selling Italian food and pasties out of her own home, and then efficiently made that dream a reality.

Nora never had a driver's license. Sure, she drove sometimes, and was also caught, but she never found the time to go down to the DMV and make things legal. Eventually, she found herself at the whim of other family members for any and all errands that needed to be run by car.

I have my own theories regarding her stubbornness to defy the system. I used to wonder how my grandmother, a survivor, an entrepreneur could tolerate *not* being able use the car when necessary. Now I think it was subconsciously planned along. It was her way of maintaining this steady swarm of followers. They'd circle "her highness" loyally awaiting individual instructions.

And yes, she did meet Fritz at the roller rink when she was fourteen. The common rumor is he danced like Fred Astaire (on wheels) and looked just like Dean Martin (that part I can attest to from photos). He was nineteen, and with my grandmother being her own original version of a Hollywood starlet, I can't help but believe their chronically re-spun tale of *Love at First Sight*.

On the nights Nora couldn't go skating and Fritz was off work, he would walk (come rain, sleet, or snow) over two miles to sit on a swing on her parents' front porch. John, Nora's dad, would eventually poke his head out the door as the signal for Fritz to hightail it home. This routine lasted over two years.

I recently took Gram to this very cool coffee shop we have in town, The Moose Jackson Café. Her response upon entering the parking lot was, "This isn't a coffee shop. That's the old North Star Hotel. This is where your grandfather took my virginity."

Good to know, Gram, good to know.

And she actually disputed the existence of the coffee shop, even as we walked in and ordered lattés. "Your grandfather and I had sex right in this very spot," she insisted. "And that was all it took, too ... the one time."

Seriously, Gram. Don't hold back. Do you want whipped cream on that latté?

Which leads me right back to 1937 ...

So five months after the encounter at the old North Star Hotel, Nora was piling on the pounds quite specifically.

"Nora? *Nora?* You better get that man of yours down to Saint Mary's and have him marry you. You're running out of time, Nora," ordered the old neighbor lady in the white house to the right of them.

Nora took heed and informed Fritz of her "condition." The following day, they dashed down to St. Mary St. Joseph Catholic Church and were wed on the spot. The only witness was the old neighbor lady in the white house to the left of them. She hustled home and promptly announced their unplanned antics to Nora's parents before she and Fritz made it onto the front porch.

Fortunately, John and Mary had a real soft spot for Fritz and moved him in pronto. And so the young couple officially began their life together.

Five years beyond that, late on the fourth of July—a night that was still buzzing with celebration—a very pregnant Nora received a single direct order from Fritz's father, Tatone. "Nora," he demanded, "Get your butt upstairs before you give birth to that baby on the lawn! I'll send Fritzie for the doctor!"

Fritz dashed from pub to pub in search of the doctor.

Meanwhile, Nora waddled up the stairs to her eight by ten room, propped a pillow between her back and the headboard, and within a few effortless minutes gave birth to a beautiful ten-pound baby boy. She was completely alone and utterly at peace as she swaddled the new baby in wet sheets and cradled him in her arms.

Her water broke as her body told her to "push" and that was it, she recalls. She said he came out clean and big and perfectly beautiful—like a two-month-old baby. The newborn had black hair, a bright round face, and spectacular inquisitive dark eyes. It was July 5, 1943.

The doctor did arrive—tipsy. He cut the cord and gave the new baby "the once over."

About one week later, one of the many young grandkids parading about the McMahon/Cerasoli dwelling pointed to the newest addition and announced, "Dickie. Let's call him Dickie."

Gram said she hadn't given it a second thought, but "Dickie" sounded good. "After all," she reasoned, "He ought to have a name, right?" And she stated the rhetorical question with pointed justification as if she were trying to convince a panel of judges who'd be apt to disagree.

So after one week in the world, my father was legally named, Richard Terry Cerasoli.

And somewhere between all that something else happened, too.

Somewhere between 1938 and 1943

Nora took in about thirteen dollars a week working in the clothing department at Montgomery Ward. Fritz didn't make much more driving truck for the city. Nora's twelve-year-old sister helped them around the house as much as she could. The house had been divided. Nora's parents lived downstairs, and Fritz and Nora rented the upstairs from them for forty dollars a month. Fritz had tried joining the Army, but was denied entry due to a medical condition. There wasn't a lot of work out there for folk like them in the late 1930s, especially in this small northern mining town. They were downright broke. They rationed food, heat, clothing, and owned neither their home nor a car. Or in Gram's frank words, "We didn't have a pot to piss in."

And then she became pregnant—again.

They were told about this man not too far out of town, a doctor who helped "people like them." They found this man. And feeling desperate and without choice, they trusted him (if you're picturing that scene from *Dirty Dancing*, picture again).

This doctor took what he referred to as "a little gold coin" and inserted it into her cervix. Then he told Nora, "Go home and forget about it." He said, "Everything will be okay now. You have nothing more to worry about."

And that was that.

She went home ... and they forgot about it.

Several months passed.

Then one evening Nora was preparing dinner when she experienced sudden and severe abdominal cramping. She looked down and saw blood running down both legs. She dropped to the floor. Slowly, she managed to crawl into the bathroom. With extreme effort she pulled herself up and onto the toilet. After what felt like an eternity—what felt like death—the pain subsided and the bleeding ceased. Nora wiped the sweat and tears from her face, then used the counter as a stabilizer and stood up. The toilet was filled with blood and tissue and something else. There inside the murky crimson water was a tiny baby cradled by the bowl. She instinctively reached down and delicately picked up the inanimate creature. The baby wasn't much bigger than the length of her hand and lacked for life. That much was certain. Nora gazed bewildered, and then attentively began counting ten fingers and ten toes.

When Fritz eventually came home, Nora showed him the miniature baby girl wrapped in a towel she held tight to her body. After agonizing deliberation, they decided together to put her delicately into a cigar box, have their own private ceremony, and bury her. They cried and held onto each other as they said a special prayer. And then they closed the door on this tragic, unimaginable event and hoped like hell that one day God would find it in his heart to forgive them.

I learned of this on one of our many walks through the Arizona desert in the spring of 1988.

"Then Dickie was born, and after that it was just a series of female issues. Bleeding, I was always bleeding." And she went on, "Some days I couldn't even walk and your grandfather would carry me up and down the stairs just so I could spend time with the family. I couldn't go to work. I could barely take care of my children."

The hemorrhaging eventually led to emergency surgery: A five-pound tumor was removed from her uterus. Along with that tumor they took the entire uterus, her fallopian tubes, and both ovaries. They said it was cancer. They said "they got it all." They said "she was fine."

She *was* fine now, except *they* had taken everything. My grandmother was left without any way for her body to produce a single female hormone. She was alive, but no longer a woman. That's how she phrased it. She called herself an "It," and stated it like a black-and-white fact absent of subjectivity or self-pity.

I think of this story often—the harshness of their reality— and hurt for both her and my grandfather. Their desperation, innocence, ignorance, fear, and complete lack of choice far exceeded anything I've personally had to endure. She was about twenty. How could God play such a cruel joke on such a perfect person, my grandmother, Nora Jo?

And then I try over and over to imagine what it might be like to be without *my* womanhood, but I cannot. I cannot imagine living without the possibility of ever experiencing love on a sexual level.

I often think we "women" like to think of sex as a *mental thing*. We rave about the importance of foreplay, a nice dinner, bottle of wine, cuddling, good conversation. Great abs do it for some. *Whatever*. What if all the great abs and good conversation in the world (plus a phenomenal foot massage and a pricey bottle of pinot) did nothing more than allow you, on solely a cerebral level, to appreciate massages, wine, abs, and good conversation? It sounds dreadfully boring and unbearably agonizing all at the same time.

She was twenty-four years old when the hysterectomy took "the woman" right out of her. I was busy downing two dollar margaritas with the-beau-of-the-moment after a night of waiting tables or performing in a play. And I was dreaming of L.A., the place where my life would truly begin. I wasn't worried about babies, or cancer, or if I could afford a dozen "uncracked" eggs. And I was about to purchase my sixth car, a nice looking Honda Accord which would drive me safely to the city where my dreams were just 'awaiting. I wasn't carting kids around (illegally) in an old, used, black Chevy that took my husband and me five years worth of penny-saving to purchase.

I sometimes wonder if this tale remains, along with a handful of tiresome others, in the shadows of her dying memories. Does it silently haunt her? But I'll never know because I'll never ask. Just as I work consciously to *never* mention my father's name, I can't imagine hurting her with questions regarding the mistakes and misfortunes of her past.

Her final admission during that particularly revealing desert jaunt some twenty-odd years ago was that she linked all these experiences collectively and accepted the outcome as the grand result. So my grandmother believed in "an eye for an eye," or in "karma" (even though that term is foreign to her). I don't know what happened to "ask and you shall receive," or "seek forgiveness and it shall be granted?" She was a diehard Catholic. I get that. Yet how come she never felt like she deserved forgiveness for being a victim of circumstance in a world without choice?

Some days, she suffered from this strange and cruel punishment that stole her sexuality, but mostly she hurt for Fritz. He was the man who had to live his life with the woman who was no longer a woman.

"He was the real victim," she ultimately admitted. "Because it was after all, my big idea to go find the man with *the little gold coin.*"

"All I have to live for is beer.
My New Year's resolution?
Drink more beer!"

Nora Jo
New Year's Eve, 2008

Blue Christmas

JOY TO THE WORLD AND BLAH BLAH BLAH. It's nearing that time of year again when the entire planet fakes "jolly." And that long-standing rumor about suicide rates rising exponentially resurfaces like candy canes, eggnog, and *Miracle on 42nd Street.* Anxiety and stress levels shoot through the roof, which makes even the most normal of families (whoever they are) a little bit frantic. There's pressure to cook, clean, shop, travel, and spread your freaking Christmas cheer with a smashing grin from ear to ear. It's down-right exhausting. In truth, "The Christmas Blues" aren't a myth, but statistically people don't off themselves any more during the holidays than they do on any given Monday. I just researched those stats and hope that makes some of you feel better (insert smiley face). They do lose track of their schedules though and gain weight, drink more, and sleep less. And for Gram, this was tough—a change in her environment. People popping in unexpectedly made her nervous. Presents, noise, chaos like kids running around wildly really shook her up. She was either confused and mad or just plain sad.

Pete and I have Jazz and Brock—two spectacular excuses to celebrate and enjoy the season. That was a no-brainer. But Gram sat in her rocker worrying, fidgeting, and filling up much of her time (which was all considered "free" at this point) with an extra dose of tears and beers. She dreaded everything that went along with the holidays. But most particularly, like my mother, she dreaded knowing she'd be spending them without her significant other. The great grandchildren were a God-given distraction, but they didn't fill the void of a deceased lifelong companion.

In addition to the grim loneliness that emanated almost visibly from her body, a high anxiety kept her heart in knots and escalated the symptoms of her illness. I was beginning to feel like Shirley MacClaine in that I swear I could see a heavy gray aura trailing Gram about the house. She slept less, senselessly chattered more, and misplaced everything—hearing aids, glasses, coffee, money, jewelry, shoes, and the list went on. She irrationally started squirreling away both food and beverage in drawers as if planning for the Second Coming. Nora Jo understood that people were going to be wandering about the house, and she was cognizant enough to discern that she wasn't going to recognize these people. Yet had enough memory left to know she was supposed to, but not enough to take that one step further and deduct she should trust them. It gave her a solid, steady fear which she covered poorly and practically nurtured by creating a dramatic and overt "indifference" about the holidays.

It gave me a whole new part-time job. One I wasn't too excited about. I had enough jobs. Plus, I'm a big fat weather baby and "zero with a chance of flurries" didn't exactly make me do jumping jacks. (Actually, nothing makes me do jumping jacks. Since giving birth to Jazz, I pee when I do jumping jacks.)

So, as cold as this will sound (truly, no pun intended), I wanted nothing more than to steer clear of Gram. She was blue, I was blue. And blue-times-two made for, well, a lotta "blue" in what was supposed to be a white Christmas. I mean, that's what we're supposed to be dreaming about, right? White. But there was no avoiding her. My position as caregiver and hers as patient made that pretty clear. There'd be no avoiding Gram this holiday season, not if I was going to play my role. And she had certainly mastered hers. Stepping up to the plate was my only choice.

So, aside from dishing out constant consolation, I also became a spy. There was nothing exciting or double-0-seven about it. I didn't have a nifty switchblade that housed truth serum and suction cups. Not that I wouldn't be doing any interrogating or wanting to climb the walls, but no one had supplied me with a "kit." My eyes, my ears, and my below-average sense of smell were my weapons. I was Agent Lisa, in charge of perishables. I reclaimed a row of Fig Newtons from her underwear drawer. I smelled apples while I was picking out undergarments for after her shower. They smelled like apples for some reason, and sure enough, there was an open row of them buried beneath a dozen granny-panties. A piece of lemon meringue pie wrapped in a napkin was stashed in a sleeveless blouse in the top drawer. Don't ask me why I looked in there. But thankfully I did before, well, sleeveless blouse season. Her sock drawer was the designated holder of anything chocolate—from mints to cookies to individually wrapped pieces to tiny, shiny boxes and her token Snickers bars. They were hidden about and inside the socks. As for her beer, she may not have actually upped her alcohol intake like I had imagined. Because over the month of December, I must have discovered somewhere in the ballpark of a case of it scattered throughout her bedroom. This was starting to feel like an Easter egg hunt. Except with an Easter egg hunt, even if it was at Grandma's, you knew you weren't going to have to rummage through her panties to find that pretty pink egg you'd colored the day before. The beer cans were rolled into sweaters, hidden between piles of perfectly folded flannel nightgowns, stuffed inside purses that were jammed under sweaters, peeking out of her winter boots, et cetera. I also found a half dozen animal crackers stuffed in the drawer where all greeting cards received since 1965 had apparently taken up residence. They lay there crowded, yellowing, and smelling like old books—the cards, not the crackers. I put Jazz on trial for that one. And after heavy duty cross-examining and permission to treat the witness "hostile," she 'fessed up to the crime, stating, "Come on, Mama, I was just messing with G.G."

"Jazz, you don't need to mess with G.G. She does that all on her own. She's losing her memory."

"I thought it would be funny."

"You can already outrun her, out talk her, and outwit her. Isn't that enough?"

"I like to be the winner. The winner!"

"Jazz, this isn't a contest. She's a ninety-year-old woman. Pick on someone your own size. Or not at all. Allow me to rephrase that. Don't pick on anyone at all."

"But, Mama, it was a little bit funny."

"Jazz, it's not nice. And they're animal crackers. G.G. doesn't even eat animal crackers. That was the dead giveaway."

"You mean I should hide something G.G. likes like chicken or beer or chicken? She loves chicken! And beer!"

"Do not stash anything in this room, understand?"

Jazz gazed up at me. She understood. I wasn't convinced she wasn't still plotting, though.

"Jazz, if I find anything suspicious in here and you did it, there will be no TV for a whole day."

"No!"

"Yes. And don't yell at me."

"You're not my best mom!"

"Watch it, little lady. You want a time-out?"

"No."

It was a stare down—one of many.

"Can I go now, Mama? I'm sorry. *Pleeease?*"

"Yes."

"Okay. Bye, Mom!"

And off to *Hannah Montana* she went.

Yeah, this is the part where you all secretly judge my parenting skills (or lack thereof). When you threaten a child with the TV, it's only because they're already watching too much of it. I know that. Before the "rescue mission," it wasn't an issue. But in nine months, it's gone from a nonissue to her entertaining *other* mother. Yes, another admission. I use the TV as my babysitter. It's free. I always know where it is. It allows me to tend to G.G., and it's *somewhat* educational. I mean, her showmanship has seriously improved thanks to shows like *Hannah Montana* and *The High School Musicals*.

Despite our own private chaos, I hoped once holiday things got rolling—two weeks' worth of extra bodies floating about our house—Gram would be fine. My bro would be coming with Jen and Jakey (who was about nine months old now). Gram just loved staring at the baby. So there was that. I held onto that shred of hope.

Wow. It certainly seems like negativity is emanating from *my* body as well. I sound like a gigantic, bitter pessimist, the quintessential grinch, a hater of Christmas. But that was not the case. There are things to be adored about the holiday. Well, there's one thing: The tree. I've always loved the tree. Decorating it is like psychotherapy and an oil painting workshop all jumbled into one. Afterwards, I feel relaxed, relieved, and downright impressed with myself. And the lights! They're hypnotic, inciting a magical mood that never dulls. There is nothing ordinary about the beauty of a decorated tree. I think the only reason to take them down at all is because they're "suckers of space," and after a while you just want your space back. That and the pesky needles on the carpet and the fact that all trees eventually become fire hazards. Those are just some of the reasons I prefer artificial trees, although there's nothing "artificial" about the feelings they instill.

I put the (fake) tree up every year by Thanksgiving and leave it till at least my birthday—the end of January. Once, I left it up till Easter, but that was in high school when I lived in my parents' basement. I could sit and dream and fall asleep by the glow of my fabulous, three-foot tree. The glamorous, unique lil' creature lulled me peacefully to sleep every night. Christmas trees are also silent narrators of a family's history, which is so cool. Gram and I spent a whole day putting up the tree. She handed me every bulb, helped me choose their positioning, then we draped it with silver beads and ribbons of copper. That was a great day, maybe the best of the season.

Oh, and I love holiday music. "The Little Drummer Boy" is my all-time fave. This kid's got nothing, this little boy, except a drum. And so he plays it for the King and it turns out to be the best gift of the night. That's what Christmas is really about. And I'm not just saying that to sound all preachy and shit. I really believe that. But everyday Gram worried about gifts. It didn't matter that I showed her presents under the tree for the kids with her name attached, she couldn't remember, so over and over she obsessed about the "gift-giving" scandal that's engulfed this holiday.

Pete and I exchange "niceties" for Christmas. He gets sex or pie (yes, lemon meringue) or both if he's lucky. And I usually get a really sweet letter. We made a pact about gift-giving in the beginning. We decided presents were for the kiddies, and we've stuck to it. What a HUGE relief. But Gram's a traditionalist, and all the redundant reassurance in the world couldn't get her to believe that Christmas was going to be okay this year. She felt like the little drummer boy, as though she had nothing to give. And she felt talent-less, too.

Then Pete came up with an idea.

The day before Christmas Eve, 2008

"Nor. Nor, get your butt out of that rocker. We're making raviolis."

"What's that, Brock?"

"I'm Pete, Nor. We're making raviolis. I need you to teach me."

Pete knew how to make ravs. Gram had already taught him the year before, and the year before that.

"Oh, shit, Pete," she grumbled, rocking back and forth in an attempt to get up and out of her chair. "I can't make ravs. My back. My mind. Jesus, I can't even remember what cheese goes into the goddamned things. Let's see ... ricotta, parmesan, mozzarella, tuma."

"Look at that, lady. You did it!"

She made it out of her rocker and shuffled over to him. He put up his hand for a high five. It was totally lost on her. He swung that arm back down, though just in time for her to grab hold of his hand and confide, "And if you *really* like who you're making them for, you also add asiago. But you gotta really like those people to make the ravs *that* special."

"Well, Nor, we *are* those people."

"Then break out the asiago! And a beer while you're at it! I'm as dry as Hades in August."

It was my husband to the rescue. Always a saint and now a superhero.

This really sharp waitress recently told me as she dropped off a fantastic glass of Red Guitar wine (which she had also recommended) that by giving birth to a boy, she finally discovered what men really need.

I leaned in closely, my eyes wide with wonder.

"They need food, entertainment, and coddling. And the only thing that changes throughout the course of their lives is the type of entertainment."

So simple. So brilliant. My husband was a lover of food (one of the three). Gram was a professional cook. Pete took one of his basic needs, combined a little compassion with his innate intuitiveness, and figured out how to give Gram what she needed. He brought her back to her roots in a pinch. And the end result would fill his needs as well—the needs of his tummy.

This was good.

Pete was definitely deserving of much more than lemon meringue.

Wake up, Lisa. Wake up. He deserves some good, old-fashioned "entertainment."

Christmas Eve, 2008

Rick and his family rolled in mid-afternoon. She didn't know him again, except as The-Big-Fat-Guy-With-The-Tattoo. He really needs to ease up on the wife-beaters. Or we could consider turning down the heat. Of course, at least his title was quite specific and oddly endearing compared to the label Gram gave his wife: That Girl.

Jazz and Jake were both "The Babies." Jake's distinguishing feature wasn't that he was two-and-a-half years younger than

Jazz and of a different sex. It was that he was fat (also). And he actually was fat, I guess. He was a new baby. He was just as he was supposed to be—big, beautiful, and healthy with perfectly plump, soft limbs and intense blue eyes that created a stunning offset to his richly brown, slightly waved, cottony hair. He was mellow and smiley. He looked just like my dad, with the exception of the dramatic eye color. He brought an extra dose of "happy" to Gram and Mom. Dickie reincarnate was *in the house.*

But even with love and family all around, by New Year's Eve Gram confessed that indeed all she had to live for was beer. And along with that admission, through another endless set of intense, sincere tears, she admitted to just wanting more of it—it was the only true happiness she had left to hold on to. That's what she claimed.

It was so sad. And weird. And a little funny, too, in all honesty. I mean how many people admit to something like that? I've been running circles around this woman—bathing her, styling her hair, cutting her toenails, doing her laundry, and most importantly sitting with her and listening to her ramblings. *And all she has to live for is her next can of Busch Light?* Merry Christmas to me.

I used to love her, oh yeah,

But I had to kill her.

I used to love her ...

Oh, cut the crap it's New Year's Eve and ...

Fa la la la la, la la la la.

She was just being honest. Like Jazz. But seriously, where's my goddamned medal?

It hits me again that this job has no glory.

Gram and Gramps had thirty years together worth of happy hours. From four to seven every day, if you popped into their place, they were serving you up a cocktail. Call it crazy. Call it funny. Call it alcoholism. For them it was tradition, a way of life, she and Fritz winding down the day, celebrating each other or forgetting their worries. I had never seen either of them drunk, not while my gramps was alive. But he was no longer alive and things were different now. Difficult. Maybe the beer reminded her of "the good old days." Maybe her fixation with it helped her forget them. In any case, we curbed the habit as best we could. What we couldn't do is find it in our hearts to strip her completely of this pleasure that also happened to be dubbed an addiction. So much was already lost. She didn't get the DTs or anything if she went a few days without beer. She just got annoyed and a little bit sadder, and the latter was unbearable. So against both professional and a handful of amateur advice, we let her drink. I'm an enabler. That's the term one of the "pros" used to describe me. But this is the end of the road for Gram. It shouldn't be completely without joy, should it? What am I to take from some of this advice? That people work their entire lives only to end up old, frail, alone, widowed, confused, in pain *and beerless, too?* Is that what we're supposed to do? Am I to strip away one of her only joys? This is a very gray area that could be debated at length. But I just don't have the time. So I'll settle for the term "enabler." I'm sure to some it seems that way. But my family and I will continue to watch over Gram in the fashion we see fit— with compassion, (a dash of fear) and some good old-fashioned wit.

As I looked down at this woman who just admitted all she has to live for is beer, I found myself stumped for words.

"Happy New Year's, Gram," Rick interjected. Then he leaned down and hugged her. "It'll be okay."

"Thank you, Ricky," she responded naturally. "Ricky." She said it again, then cupped her hands around his and smiled up at him, consumed with a childlike delight.

Just like that, she knew his name.

So I fibbed a few pages back. Trimming the tree was the second ... no, actually the third best day of the season for Nora Jo. And making raviolis with Pete was her second favorite day. But dishing them out to her family on Christmas Eve as we raved on and on—that was by far the highlight of her holiday. She scooped up the praises, each one better than the last, and filed them away systematically like she was being interviewed for a job she knew she already had. In truth, Pete and I screwed up on the dough. It was tough. No one said a word. Gram got all the credit for our spectacular meal. She had purchased no actual gifts, but this was better than a "sweater." And watching her glow was more priceless than any gift card we could have received. She played her drum that night for all to hear, and it was magical. She had indeed brought her gift to the King. And, boy, did she beam.

Dementia Facts and Fiction

August, 2004

THE FOUR OF US PILED INTO THE BLUE Buick— Pete, my mom, Gram, and me. Rick and Jen had purchased their first home and we were heading downstate to see it. This was before babies and any formal diagnosis of mental illness. But, it was after Grandpa's death—just two short months and only one year after both dads, mine and Pete's (which also felt like two short months). Our lives were basically being lived and planned around distraction after distraction. My mother had bought a house a few months back, and it needed a ton of work. Distraction. Rick just bought one that needed updating, too. Another distraction. We were all heading down to spend a week there. Decidedly more distraction.

It's amazing the four of us even fit in the car after Gram packed all the "necessities" of travel. She had enough food in a series of paper bags, cardboard boxes, and even a plastic dishpan to launch her own bomb shelter. She was not a good traveler. Even in her pre-demented state, the woman grew anxious and overly cautious at the thought of this trip. So why was she going? Distraction.

It was fascinating down in Detroit watching Gram this far out of her element.

"Lisa, Sherie, come look at this!" she yelled.

We walked into the kitchen as Gram was opening up a loaf of bread. "They have twist ties down here. Well, I'll be goddamned. Twist ties in Detroit? Who'd a thought something like twist ties could make it all the way to the city? But sure as shit, here they are."

We watched in awe as she held it up to the light to inspect its authenticity.

"Pete. Pete?" she called out.

"Peter's at the store with Rick, Ma," my mother said through a series of giggles.

"Do you think he knows about the twist ties?" Gram continued.

"Well, he's got a master's degree and he traveled the world when he was in the Marines, I'm pretty sure he knows about the twist ties," I managed to interject before doubling over.

"Oh," she replied with sincere disappointment in her tone.

We curbed our hysteria as best we could.

Again, allow me to reiterate. This was before the dementia. This? This was just Gram.

Another thing that baffled her daily was the mailman. She couldn't believe Detroit had mailmen. She perched herself by the window to watch the mail get delivered all week. "He walks it right up to the box and puts it right in, just like they do in Iron

Mountain."

"Everybody gets the mail, Gram."

"Sure, sure. But how does he manage to get to *all these houses?* There must be a million of 'em."

"Well, you know, Nor, they hire a few more down here than we have up north," Pete reasoned.

"They goddamned better," Gram concurred.

At one point during dinner, Gram stood up and dropped trou(ser). She had been wearing my gramps Fruit of the Loom BVDs religiously since his death and thought it was important to tell Rick and Jen about it, about how comfortable they were. And she really wanted to show them how well they fit. During dinner. As she yanked her pants back up and we all stepped away from the table (if that's not a "meal" breaker, I don't know what is), she confessed feeling like a fool for never having tried them on while he was alive.

And that was our vacation.

You get the gist.

FACT: There are ten warning signs that send out a red alert that someone you know may have early onset dementia or Alzheimer's:

1. Short-term memory loss.

2. Confusion with time or place.

3. Changes in mood and personality.

4. Misplacing things.

5. Difficulty in performing routine tasks.

6. Withdrawal from work or social activities.

7. Decreased or poor judgment

8. Challenges in planning and solving problems.

9. Impaired speech and writing skills.

10. Loss of spatial reasoning.

Okay, so the first five warning signs sound symptomatic of many conditions, including anxiety, stress, insomnia, *motherhood*. Both pregnancy and motherhood brought dementia-like symptoms into my existence for nearly the first three years. Just when I was recovering, Gram moved in, and they started all over again. I was beginning to think it was contagious. And I was wondering if an Aricept or two might help me remember where I last left my cell phone.

FACT: Alzheimer's is the most common form of dementia. It accounts for up to seventy percent of all cases. It is a disease that has seven stages and usually lasts eight years before claiming the life of its victim. But in some instances, people have been known to live as long as twenty years. Other forms of dementia such as Vascular, Mixed and Frontotemporal (Pick's Disease) have symptoms similar to those of Alzheimer's but their path of progression is less systematic. These diseases have a tendency to hit faster, lasting three to six years, and sometimes the decline occurs in steps rather than slowly and steadily. But just like with Alzheimer's, people revert to childhood memories when the brain has lost its ability to retain anything "in the present."

Nora Jo has actually been diagnosed with both diseases. I don't know if it comes down to "a matter of opinion" or a test. A scan of her brain verified small blood vessel disease. Her earliest symptom (confusion at night) was coined "sundown syndrome" and was associated with dementia. As her disease has progressed, however, her doctors have thrown around the term "Alzheimer's." She has had an oral and written evaluation that has categorized her as a "16" on a scale of "1 to 30" with 30 being the most severe. Some doctors have gone to great lengths to explain the difference, while others have blown me off as if the terms are interchangeable. All I really know for sure is that one is a subcategory of the other. It's like if dementia were our solar system, then Alzheimer's would be Jupiter. I personally think Gram has Vascular Dementia. I notice big dips in her mental capabilities and then sudden plateaus where it seems as though she's improving for a couple of weeks. But what the hell do I know? I'm only with her twenty-four hours a day.

FACT: The biggest risk factor for developing some form of dementia is increase in age. Another high risk factor is family history.

Yikes. My people live long and get crazy. I've got "screwed" written all over me.

FACT: Eighty-four million people worldwide have some form of dementia. There is no known cure. The best treatment to date is to maintain familiarity. If that can be achieved along with companionship and a sense of purpose, chances are it will extend a person's mental capacities better than any drug currently on the market.

FACT: Over five million Americans currently suffer from Alzheimer's Disease.

FACT: Of all the people currently diagnosed with this disease, fifty percent of them still live alone. They are responsible for their own cooking, cleaning, bill paying, and personal care. Most still possess a driver's license.

I truly believe had Nora Jo been placed in a facility that specializes in dementia, she would no longer have any cognitive attachments to family or to her history. She'd be in "lockdown." The idea in most facilities is to keep these people from escaping. And it works. It efficiently locks down their bodies. Unfortunately, it does the same with their minds. But what are the choices if there is no alternative? I'm in no way knocking nursing home facilities. I'm saying with Gram, there was a choice. And she feels lucky to have had that. Despite the unpredictable behavior, she's grateful everyday. That has remained a sweet and sincere constant. Every meal is luscious, that's her "gold medal" term for all of Pete's cooking. And every pot of coffee brewed before she rises to meet the day has been done with sheer perfection, even if it's sat for hours.

As far as a sense of purpose goes, that's a very patient-specific dilemma. Gram loves folding our laundry (and we *really* love it, too). Go Gram! But, Beau? Her mind is no longer capable of taking on new duties, especially in regard to a living, breathing thing.

Folding dish towels? *Awesome.*

Small dog? *Annoying nuisance.*

FACT: Seventy percent of Alzheimer's patients are cared for at home thereby impacting the lives of millions of family members, friends and caregivers.

My grandpa Fritz grew more and more silent as this disease engulfed his mind. He somehow knew to "fake" smiles when all surrounding conversation was lost on him. He never entered into a combative stage. He wandered out at night once. That was after Gram gave him a sleeping pill. Evenings were tough because Gramps would call out in his sleep, and he'd have vivid and sometimes violent dreams. So Gram slipped him a sleeping pill to give them both some relief, and that's when he wandered out in the middle of the night in the middle of the winter. Thankfully, he was found by the police. Although he required hospitalization, his injuries were not severe. They could have been deadly. Snow still covered the ground and he hadn't thought to put on his shoes.

My mom and I would alternate sleeping there a couple nights a week to help out Gram. Other family members did what they could by day.

One night really stands out in my memory. I laid in bed across the hall from their room—pillows jammed into my ears.

"Go, Charlie! You goddamned son of a bitch! Get that Nazi! Kill 'em dead!" My gramps was seriously bellowing out these strange commands. Then he'd mimic the sounds of gunfire and start yelling all over again. "Get 'em, Charlie! Go!"

This went on all night. Until then, I'd never heard of a "Charlie."

By morning, I sat exhausted at the kitchen table while Gram went about the business of frying up breakfast as if it were just a regular morning.

"Gram, does Gramps have nightmares every night?"

"Yep. Like clockwork. Same old shit. It's him and Charlie against the world. Whoever the hell that guy is."

"Don't you think it's funny that he reverts back to World War II in his sleep?"

"Yeah, I think it's real funny—especially since he only made it as far as Milwaukee, Wisconsin. They sent him straight back to me on account of his flat feet."

No wonder she drugged him.

Gramps eventually came downstairs, clueless about all his late night dramatics. He smiled sweetly and sat in his usual chair patiently waiting for coffee. It was quite precious watching the two of them assume their roles without any regard for the illness engulfing him. But for the most part, he had stopped speaking during his waking hours, save for the occasional giggle which accompanied a series of nods.

My gram's verbal communications have decreased in quality but conversely increased in quantity. She's extremely paranoid, but that's been a lifelong trait. I'd be surprised if she wandered anywhere.

Her brain has forgotten how to tell her stomach she's "full." And she can't remember if she's eaten, so she could literally eat nonstop, if you let her. Yet she stays thin. She loves sweets now.

Never touched them in her other life. I've witnessed her eat an entire apple pie over the course of one night. And half of that was with a finger-to-mouth technique she's recently acquired. We used to scold her. Now we just spread word throughout the house in code: Gram: Fingers: Apple Pie: *Got it.*

This enigmatic disease is unique to every individual. Patterns developed through habits and throughout a person's history will carry through. They will often balloon—particularly dominant personality traits, making these individuals take on a caricature-like form of their old identity.

I've spent a considerable amount of time studying this specific illness. I'm no Ph.D. but I have intense "hands on" knowledge. I've had both grandparents to watch and care for on some level. So I have learned a thing or two. Books are a beautiful thing, but they don't replace instinct. And support is salvation—any kind, any time. Don't ever say no to that. News programs can give up-to-date information just like the Internet, but for the most part, if it's not a documentary, TV and the movies have a tendency to "romanticize" this illness. I get it. That's what TV and the movies are for— to entertain us, not necessarily prepare us.

I was channel surfing in the hopes of finding just that, some mindless entertainment when I landed upon the movie, *The Notebook*. Nicholas Sparks wrote the novel. It's a quaint little love story that tears at your heartstrings and gives the world an overview of what having Alzheimer's truly means. It was made into a hit movie. TMC was showing it and it was just beginning. The movie was very well cast and well-written. I found it to be enchanting, stirring, sexy, sweet, and tragic. It managed to portray, quite spectacularly I think, one hell of a lifelong love story. *And if* Quentin Tarantino had directed it, it might resemble something close to what "Life with Nora Jo" has been like thus far.

Chapter Seven

*"Just give me five minutes at midnight with a nice fluffy pillow ...
and you people can go back to business as usual."*

Rick
February 14, 2009

Me and My (Drunk) Shadow

It's absolutely, illegally freezing. Schools have been closed four days so far this year due to wind chill factors that dropped temperatures to more than twenty-five degrees below zero. Iron Mountain is knee-deep in ice and snow. And since the elderly don't do well with the cold and the ice and the snow, they stay indoors for fear of "breaking a hip."

February, 2009

Gram hasn't left the house in three weeks. This isn't because we haven't tried. Some days she sleeps until mid-afternoon. Other days she takes one look out the window and then looks at us like we're crazy for even suggesting an out-of-house excursion. All of the days though, she's unmistakably freezing. The fireplace, the space heater, an electric blanket, microwavable mittens ... nothing warms the woman up. Everyone in the house is either dying of heat or walking around half naked, with the exception of Jazz and me. Jazz *is* naked. And I'm freezing, too.

We're starting to mirror each other, my grandmother and I, as we hang about, wrapped in our white terry cloth robes. We've taken on a duo drag-like *signature* shuffle, too. We actually glide now—no picking up of the feet whatsoever. We don't have carpeting, and between the hard core wind chill factors outside and the mentally unstable issues inside, there's no reason to pick up our feet when we walk anymore. Part of this mirrored image effect is my fault. In addition to our robes, I bought us matching boot slippers, the poor man's version of an Ugg. And part of it's her fault: genetics. I came out bearing a pretty hefty dose of the Cerasoli DNA. My Gram and I have the same exact body types and mannerisms, and we share a lot of the same compulsions. Basically, we're a couple of hypochondriacs who both suffer from anxiety and a touch of OCD. It's fun for Pete. Except, I like things neat and clutter free. By the time I'm eighty, I'll probably be sitting on a yoga mat in the middle of an otherwise empty living room. My Gram, on the other hand, is a pack rat. Nothing is garbage to this woman. Parting with an overused Kleenex is often harder than kissing "The Baby" good-bye. So the "circle of life" in this house is Gram stockpiling as much shit as possible in her bedroom and leaving oodles of other crap lying EVERYWHERE ... and me working like a madwoman to undo her trails and stashes of trash. I guess in a way this keeps us both pretty busy. That's another trait we both have in common. We like our time to be fully occupied (or at least Gram used to).

The thing about being trapped indoors with someone who has lost all sense of purpose is that they have a tendency to glom onto yours. So if Gram's not busy antagonizing Jazz for the umpteenth time to put on socks, she's stalking me. Sometimes she'll eye me steadily from three feet away, studying me as though I were a lab rat. From dishes to decorating—there she is, in my path, one hand on a hip, the other holding a Busch Light. She's either hindering my pace or just plain creeping the crap out of me because sometimes I don't know she's there. My mind's on cleaning floors or in the throes of some kind of self-help "I think I can" mantra when— BAM—there's Gram shocking me senseless with one of her odd sayings. These are always in the third person, which somehow makes them more annoying.

She's gonna scrub down to the floorboard, that girl. She better ease up there.

Or ...

A woman's job is never done.

Or ...

Poor, poor Lisa ... that's man's work.

Or ...

That girl is gonna work herself into the grave.

Or ...

She can't lift that. Where's the men?

Who is she talking to?

One night after she had gone to bed, I turned off all the lights and then thought to check the garage door, as I didn't remember shutting it. When I walked into the dark entranceway, a shadowy form scared the bejeezus out of me.

"Oh, hi, honey," says the shadowy form of my gram like it's morning time, like the lights are actually on, or like she's NOT making her way into a dark garage for no good reason.

A bloodcurdling scream exploded from my lips as I sprang into the air. I'm pretty sure I managed to throw some kind of manic kickboxing move directly at her head.

"I'm sorry, honey, did I scare you?" she questioned, just as coolly and nonchalantly as her first comment.

Are you kidding me?

I grabbed my heart. *Okay, good. It's still inside my body.* Then I fell flat across the kitchen counter. "Gram! What? Are? You? Doing?" Each word came out as its own sentence.

"I was thirsty. I'm dry."

"You were going into the garage."

"I was just looking."

"Maybe a light next time? Turn on a light."

"Okay, sweetheart, I sure will. Goodnight, dear. I love you."

"Love you, too."

Ugh.

The good news is she still had a nose. And to get weird and look on the brighter side of life, at least I now knew my reaction if faced with an intruder. There'd be an attempted ass-kicking if I didn't die of a heart attack first. So that was reassuring.

What wasn't reassuring was the I-don't-give-a-shit mood that had come over me during this eleven-month carnival ride. It wasn't just the weather, it wasn't just Gram. There was an odd indifference slithering about my insides and I didn't care for it one bit. A plan to rid myself of this twitchy case of the doldrums needed to be set in action. I immediately started weaning myself from Paxil, started practicing yoga at least three days a week, and made a doctor's appointment with a neurologist regarding my headaches.

Three Weeks Later

"What you have is something we like to call SAD or Seasonal Affective Disorder. You shouldn't be weaning yourself of any medication on your own. The problem is your body has adapted to the Paxil. We need to double the dose, not take you off of it. And the headaches are both structural and stress related, so let's continue to cope with those through medication and exercise." She stated oh, so pleasantly.

It's been twenty-five below for forty days in a row and the sun hasn't shown its shiny face since before the holidays ... and I'm SAD? Of course, I'm SAD! But this is my diagnosis? The fact that this is a diagnosis at all is ludicrous. You know what I think? It's a Shitty Ass Day. And so was yesterday, it was SAD, too. And tomorrow's gonna be another Shitty Ass Day. And if that doesn't piss you off or make you SAD, maybe you need some meds.

I didn't say all that. I might have, but found myself still trapped in that I-don't-give-a-shit mood and wasn't up for arguing. So she doubled my prescription and then I crumpled it up and bounced it off the wall and into the garbage can on the way out. *Two points.*

Rick blew back into town a week later to help Pete and me

tile twelve hundred square feet of basement. We put the house on the market like the rest of the planet. We were concerned about Pete getting pink-slipped and needed the house to look staged by spring.

Pete was busy at school all day and also with coaching. Although I was still doing real estate, it had basically become a "volunteer" job, so Rick coming in saved everyone. He had "work" for a couple of weeks. Pete got a break from having to pull off this basement with just me. And I got real, live, adult interaction, which had to be better than a triple dose of Paxil. In any case, it did the trick.

Rick noticed a considerable decline with Gram since Christmas. Aside from the expected "name" and "relationship" confusion, her redundancy had reached a new high.

"Good morning, Leonard."

"Hey, Gram. It's afternoon. And I'm Rick."

"Oh, right. Rick. I'm the Grandma."

"I know, Gram. I'm your grandson."

"I thought you looked familiar. I'm going to make myself a cup of coffee. Do you want one?"

"You're coffee's on the kitchen table, Gram. And you have one in the microwave, too. I'll get that one for you."

Rick reheats the coffee and sets it down on the table, exchanging it out for the old one.

"Thank you, Brock."

"I'm Rick, Gram."

"Right. Now how do I know you? Do you live here?"

"No, Gram. I'm Rick. I live in Detroit."

"I'm just visiting, too. I'm the Grandma."

It was a mind-numbing experience for him, to say the least. It's harder to weave in and out of this place than it is to just live here, I'll tell you that much.

In addition to the daily vaudevillian sock routine she had established with Jazz, she would also break out this old photo album and question the identity of everyone in it. This sounds healthy and productive in theory, but in reality some of the people were dead and that put her in a legitimate panic, and others just didn't come around like they used to. Dementia is a strange beast. It's hard on people. Some can't conceptualize it. We've often heard, *What's the point? It's not like she'll remember if I come.* Sure, she won't remember, but if you take the time to visit, it'll make her so happy for the moment. And that's the point. But sometimes I'm even one of those people. I've ducked and dodged Gram. There have been occasions when "one night to myself" is honestly required to reenergize. So I've hidden away with a good book for a couple of hours and then sneaked back into my "post" in the living room. Once the lie, *I had just gone to the bathroom,* flew right out of my mouth. I know. Horrible. But it's a strange and overwhelming thing. Dementia is a *can or can't do* illness. It's not for everybody. So we love any and all visitors and will take 'em whenever we get 'em. No questions asked.

Anyway, there's Rick and Gram with the family photo album. "That's So-n-So, Gram, with you and Gramps in your backyard." He said.

Then Gram would point to another person.

"Nope. I've never seen that person before in my life."

Then she'd flip the page and look to Rick for more answers.

"Oh, that's So-n-So at your eightieth birthday party."

Then she'd smile and move to the next person.

"Nope. I've never seen that person before in my life."

I watched in envious awe. Why hadn't I thought of that?

When the photo album extravaganza finally came to a close, Gram got up, hugged Rick and returned the book to some safe refuge, because it hasn't been seen since.

Then Rick approached me with a bit of a swagger, cracked his knuckles, and said, "There you go, Lis. I just wiped out half the family. That's one problem solved."

"Thank you, Rick. That was amazing. I am truly in awe of you right now."

"I'm in awe of you. And Pete. And Brock. And Jazz. I don't know how you people do this day in and day out."

"You would, too, if you were here."

"Yeah, sure I would. But I'm not here." Then he shook his head and uttered, "Shit."

He was right. This was the hardest winter of our lives. Rick's visit was a lifesaver. So was Ashton Kutcher, by the way.

There's only so much CNN one household can handle. Ashton recurring on *Larry King Live* during his Facebook challenge (or was it Twitter?), saved lives here at the Weaver's. And so did the eighth season of *American Idol*. We never would have lived through February without that two-night-per-week distraction.

Other than *American Idol* and CNN, the only show Gram was interested in watching was *Curb Your Enthusiasm*. Go figure, right? Well, I thought about it and came up with a theory. When we were little and spent the night with her and Gramps, they were either tuned into *The Lawrence Welk Show* or *Benny Hill*. So *American Idol* is a modern day *Lawrence Welk Show* of sorts, and Larry David equals Benny Hill. Is anybody with me?

By spring we had tallied up a healthy handful of God and/or Hollywood-sent diversions that had gotten us through winter.

And just maybe, we were all starting to get the swing of this thing, too.

*"Your Gram is standing stark naked in OUR
bathroom this time: Do you think maybe it's a sign?"*

Pete
A date he's blocked permanently from memory

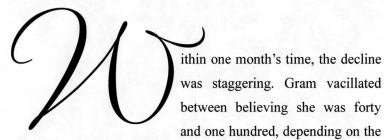

Happy Birthday
to Who?

Within one month's time, the decline was staggering. Gram vacillated between believing she was forty and one hundred, depending on the time of day and the number of beers ingested. By sundown, like clockwork, she was convinced she was Jazzy's mommy. Like a fool, I used logic to persuade her otherwise. I talked about the age gap and how women can't get pregnant after menopause. I might as well have been speaking Swahili. Some other things were happening, too.

If I left the room for any reason, my return was received as a near-reunion. That is, if they weren't trailing me. Between Jazz, my Gram and Beau, I haven't peed alone since the summer of '05. But in less than a year, Nora Jo's memory went from being like Drew Barrymore's in *Fifty First Dates* to just like Ten Second

Guy's in *Fifty First Dates*. If you haven't seen the flick, go rent it. It's worth it just to get the idea.

She's virtually lost track of time. The clock I've purposely placed in her bedroom is as neglected by her eyes and mind as the calendar hanging next to it. She can tell time now only by looking at the stove, which gets pretty interesting. 395 to her means it's five minutes till *Oprah*. For us it means it's time to throw in the pizza.

Day and night have become indistinguishable concepts. She dresses at three o'clock in the morning, then barges into our room and flips on the lights. These occurrences have been happening with more frequency. As hard as I want to, I do not react pleasantly to them.

And even though she's dead-set on establishing parental control over her most precious commodity, Jazz, she often can't recall her name or discern if she's a boy or a girl. And most days she picks endless quarrels with her over these two topics. This is when Jazz is drilled with a series of absurd questions that she answers defensively because they bug her (just like they used to bug me before I worked to adapt).

It felt much less like a steady mental decline and much more like Gram's brain took a leap off of a cliff from our vantage point. It was scary. I wanted my gram back—even the one from two months ago was looking pretty good.

It didn't seem like that was going to happen, though.

It was March, and we turned focus to her upcoming birthday. We talked about it incessantly like she was Jazz. It was so stupid. I don't even look forward to my own birthdays anymore, why would

Gram get all excited about hers? She wasn't turning five. That much she knew. What happened, instead, is we created confusion of mass proportion amongst her cliff diving gray matter. Every day started turning into her birthday. And if she didn't wake up ready to celebrate it, she was planning it for the following day ... and telling anyone who'd listen.

We have celebrated her birthday four times this year. Once she turned one hundred. She got on that kick steady for about two weeks. We finally broke down and had a party. My mom made lemon bars and everybody sang. Jazz, who loves a party, found it quite unfair that G.G. gets so many birthdays compared to her "one," but sang along nonetheless. She only reminded G.G. three or four times that evening that it wasn't really her birthday.

On the actual date, some family blew in with gifts and spirits. It was a surprise and it was amazing and, for some inconceivable reason, Gram was as clear and clairvoyant as a goddamned psychic. They reminisced for hours. She told stories of days gone by with startling accuracy. She laughed at their jokes, loved their presents, and capped off the night with an endless string of hugs, kisses, and "I love yous." That day in particular *really* pissed me off.

Seriously, Gram—you've been referring to my kid as "that little boy" for weeks now. Plus around midnight you wander around the house crying and searching for *your* little boy or you get fully dressed and pop in on us. You've been stashing perishables in your underwear drawer since Christmas and ... well ... some relatives come by that you haven't seen in six months and suddenly you've got a photographic memory? I swear if you would have asked her about the quadratic equation she would have pulled the term "square root" right out of her ass.

This is just another "life isn't fair" moment. Dementia has a lovely habit of pointing out a lot of those.

No, really, I was happy for her and, once I got over myself, it was a relief. That was the slit of light I'd been searching for throughout this long, cold winter. She dipped back up from her plunge. How long will it last? Who knows. But I just witnessed it, so it was real. She couldn't fake it. And she surely wasn't faking all the other crazy crap. No one not behind bars is that good. And there was nothing disingenuous about this woman. Ever.

August, 1985

There we were, near tears, being torn apart by a can of Alberto VO5.

My parents had put their house up for sale. My father had purchased land and was going to build his dream home in the woods, just a couple miles from town. The house wasn't on the market long when it sold. He got a great offer, which meant we were out of there. The land he purchased was still vacant, so the family got split between grandparents until the house was finished. My mom's mother took half of us, and Gram and Gramps took the other half. This had to be the coolest year of my adolescence. Not only was I blocks from my new high school and tons of other action, but I was living with the only two people that have never been mad at me in their entire lives.

Gram used to watch me when I was a tiny little tot. She boasted about me crying like hell every time Mom came to pick me up after work. That was her claim to fame: my utter adoration for her.

I don't remember any of that. But I imagine some of the same emotions were brewing beneath the surface as my gram and I faced off, separated only by a bottle of Alberto VO5.

You see, I had been living with them for a year now. The house took about eight months to build. Everyone else moved into the new place back in the spring. You do the math. I was so happy living with my grandparents, moving back home wasn't even being entertained. Happy is not even the word. Exuberant. I'm not saying we didn't hit a glitch or two. I was a bit of a teen wild child and got into trouble here and there on the weekends. But those two people were so much fun to be around, they often were my "Friday night." Their stories were priceless. The food was to die for. They did nothing but love me nonstop and they watched great TV. We made great memories together. I didn't lose my virginity at their house or anything like that, but I'm pretty certain I found out "who shot J.R." while sitting between them on their new velvety beige floral printed couch.

My friends would come over after school and Gram would stuff our faces (this was back when high school girls still ate). Then my boyfriend would pop by around dinner, hook himself up with a meal, and off we'd go to study or make out.

It wasn't just me. Everybody adored them. Everybody except my mom and dad who were growing increasingly perturbed. They wanted me to move home. But they wanted it to happen of my own volition. Basically, they wanted me to want to move home. Where was their logic? I was fifteen. *Logic?*

My father had an unbreakable respect for his parents, and my mother had been calling them "Mom" and "Dad" since she was seventeen. There was no way they were going to fight with them over me, or over anything. They just stopped coming over every day and called less frequently. They were employing a very mild version of "the silent treatment." It was genius. And it worked. *Dammit.*

And so there we were ...

An hour prior to *The Alberto VO5 Incident of 1985*, I was politely informed by Gram that it was time to pack my bags and move out. The parental figures would be picking me up shortly. My jaw hit the floor and the waterworks weren't far behind.

Gram sat me on the bed and pulled me in close. This wasn't to console. This was to confide, like girlfriends do. "It's not us, sweetheart. We want you to stay. Shit, live here till you're eighty. Daddy and I, we love having you here. But it's them—your parents. They're no longer speaking to us. And we like them. We like it when they talk to us. So you gotta pack it up. We can't break up the family over this. And we'll still see each other everyday."

This sucked.

For Gram's sake, I pulled myself together. It was a trap and we were both its victims. I mean, she was still on my team, and as a fellow teammate I had to be strong.

I started packing. That part was easy. Most of my stuff was on the floor anyway. It took like twenty minutes and I maintained my cool the entire time. Then she came in with that damned can of hairspray.

I can't even remember what the hell I was using on my "do"

before moving in with Gram. It was probably something cheap and nasty like Aqua Net. All of a sudden, here I am with the g-parents, and Gram has opened both my eyes and my mid-1980s hairdo to the beauty of Alberto VO5. We went through cans of that shit faster than spaghetti, and we ate that for breakfast sometimes. My hair had never looked better. *Or bigger.*

"Here, honey," Gram said, holding the can out in front of me. "I want you to have this."

My fingers wrapped around it right below hers, but neither one of us held on tight enough for the other to let go. "No, Gram. I couldn't. That's your last bottle."

"I know, I know. But I want you to have it, sweetheart." She nudged it a bit. "Take it."

"I can't take your last bottle."

"I'm telling you, honey," she grew flush and paused, then recovered just barely so she could finish her sentence. "I really want you to have it."

And that is when tears exploded from my eyes. I am sobbing. I'm a complete mess. I mean, my hair still looked fabulous, but the rest of me was mush. And so was Gram. She dropped the can of hairspray into my open suitcase and pulled me in for one of the most heartfelt hugs ever. And she was sobbing, too. Some team player I am.

"It's okay, honey. We're still gonna see each other. Every day. I promise." She wiped at her tears with freshly manicured nails, then took the corner of her apron to try and clean me up. My tears required more mopping than swatting.

"Jesus," she added, "we could walk to each other's damned

houses if we had to. Can't be more than a couple of miles?"

It was true. Our houses were exactly two miles away from each other.

We got ourselves together by the time my mom and dad arrived. And with as much grace as an angry, hormonally unsound, fifteen-year-old girl could possibly muster, I said my good-byes and got into their ride.

I took up walking as a genuine form of exercise that very next day.

And Gram was right. Two miles wasn't so far.

Chapter Nine

"Mom! G.G.'s trying to make me wear socks again!"

Jazzlyn Jo
Every single day of
September, October, November, December, January,
February, March, April and May.

Just the Two of Us

September, 2003

That was our wedding song: "Just the Two of Us." But it was never really just the two of us. Pete had Brock. I was living with my mom. So it was, with our fathers recently deceased, that it seemed perfectly logical when Mom suggested we all cohabitate for the first year. Overall, it worked out pretty well. Mom and I never fought, and we worked like a team around the house. Brock learned how to make his bed *and* do laundry (he'll thank me someday, I know it). Also, it kind of felt like Pete and I were back in high school, except "my boyfriend" was allowed to sleep over. *So it was, like, you know, I had, like, the coolest Mom on, like, the planet. You know?* Of course, we fought like couples do, but that too took on an amusing yet daft high school vibe.

One night, we were getting ready to go to dinner with friends and I asked him how my pants looked. The next second, I was running down the hall screaming, "Mom! Pete said my ass looks fat!"

"Oh, sweetheart, your butt could never look fat." My mother brushed off his insult with a wave of the hand and a silly grin.

"Sher, I never said that!" Pete retorts as he barrels into the kitchen. "I said I didn't love the pants. I didn't say anything about her ass, Sher." Then he turns to me. "You know I love your ass. And that's why I think you should be putting it in better pants. I'm actually sticking up for your ass here, if you stop to think about it."

It's no wonder my mother bought a fixer-upper.

But Pete was great with her. He was the "shoulder" upon which she wept regularly. There was still a living, breathing "man" in the house. He wasn't my dad, but he sure as hell was *all guy*—a real guy's guy—just as my dad was. He was instrumental in getting her through that first year. At some point, we decided that if we still liked each other by year's end, we'd try to have a baby. Surprisingly, we did (still like each other). So I broke out a calendar, *drank the water*, stood on my head, and Jazz was born June 1, 2005.

She wasn't quite two when we started noticing disconcerting behavioral issues with Gram. Jazz wasn't sleeping through the night yet, although she had long since mastered the art of walking, talking, dressing, and had fully potty-trained herself. But we were still breast-feeding. What can I say? We fancy ourselves very European (at least, that's my excuse). We lived a very liberal yet old school or "old country" lifestyle, whatever you want to call it. Anyway, let's call it "European." That way it sounds worldly and sophisticated. But I was mostly still breast-feeding because it was easy and the books (the thirty-five I read on pregnancy and parenting) all told me it was beneficial until she was two.

It started out as an ordinary day in April of 2007, until I walked in on the near-breast-feeding incident. *And if I walked in on it ...* we can all deduct it wasn't my breast that was about to do the feeding. That was one of the first triggers that something was happening.

Gram was also evolving into an impatient person with a series of unwarranted or fabricated frustrations. In the past, I would have never described her that way. We watched this for a year before braving the unknown and moving her in.

Jazz

I think if it were possible for me to read minds, the closest I'll ever come is reading my Jazzy's. This change has been trying on her. Her life is off, different, and compromised compared to the lives of most of her friends. Because I believe in her resilient spirit and know her like no other, I know that she'll survive it, too.

We named her after Pete's dad, Jack. He played the sax in a jazz band when he was younger, and he dated a former jazz singer as an adult. Jazz was the music that resonated throughout his world. It's funny when you choose a name for someone and then their personality coils and climbs right around it like vines on an old stone wall. I can't imagine my little girl being named anything else. She's smart, sassy, high energy, funny, unpredictable, sweet, and soothing. She's all that "Jazz." Fortunately, moving in her Great Grandmother didn't put any one of her dynamic character traits on pause, but in contrast, it's served to amplify a few.

Prior to this, she was a lot like an only child. With over ten years between her and Brock, they didn't have much to fight about outside of their favorite food, "strawberries." If not for frequent squabbles over the last strawberry in the basket, their relationship would be perfect. More like mentor-child than brother-sister. But with Gram, Jazz finally had the annoying little sister she never asked for. And as the months staggered on and my tolerance level steadily decreased, I relied more and more on my young daughter to interact with her unpredictable new "sister." I've had family members and even a doctor tell me this isn't fair. They've said, "Jazz doesn't deserve to be witness to the unraveling of your grandmother. The bickering, the antagonizing—it's not fair to a little girl."

Their perspective is quite perceptive, yet I politely disagree with it. Mostly because life isn't fair. *And?*

Jazzy's space has been invaded. She has three people watching over her now. Some of us are bossier than others, some of us try to get her to wear "socks" more than others, and some of us carry a constant and unhealthy obsession regarding her safety and identity. Even when G.G. truly believes she's Jazz's mama, they argue more like sisters, with Jazz being the older and more cunning of the two.

But Jazz is Nora Jo's salvation. Whether she's excited about the role or not, she is the reason this woman has any will to go on. As mentioned earlier, I bought the woman a poodle (brain surgeon that I am). Meanwhile, what truly gets her out of bed "midday" isn't the poodle but rather magic—the magic of Jazz. It's a lot for a child. But don't we all feel that way about our children? They are born and suddenly our existence changes planes. We move into this zone where "Love" and "Risk" are forever escalated and "Purpose" no longer goes on vacation. It's right there, in your face, everyday.

And knowing your grandparents on an intimate level is precious and priceless. It molds you into a more compassionate, understanding adult. I mean, that's how we all got here in the first place. This stranger-than-fiction scenario has all spun from my grandmother, Nora Jo, playing a vital role in my life as a girl and as a woman.

So Jazz complains and sticks out her tongue and plays tricks and games. But she also helps me get Gram in and out of the shower, and is the first to race and tell me if G.G. looks sick. She grabs Gram's walker if she can't get up from her rocker, and she has become designated "door holder," a job she enjoys and brags about. How is this detrimental to the development of my child?

Most people see "the big picture." They are not there for the kiss that's blown across the room before bedtime or the "coloring contests" or the praise Jazz receives, even after the thirtieth somersault when the rest of us have long since moved on to something more stimulating.

While piling groceries into the Jeep the other day, we watched a very old woman get hoisted out of a car and plopped down into a wheelchair. Then her daughter or whoever pushed her watchfully across the parking lot. With her head permanently affixed in a downward position, the fragile creature looked hardly conscious, barely alive. I buckled Jazz in and we drove in silence for about a minute.

"Mama," Jazz finally whispered.

"Yes, lovey."

"Don't be mad."

"I'm not mad. What's up?"

"I hope G.G. dies before she has to be in that chair."

I smiled back at her through the rearview mirror. "I'm not mad, honey."

"I want G.G. to have one more birthday cause it's so much fun to have a birthday party. Then I hope she dies and goes to be in Heaven before she has to be in that chair. I do not like that chair."

"I don't like that chair either, Jazz. That's sweet, Jazz, what you're saying. I'm not mad. What you're saying is really, really sweet, my love."

That was the mind of my daughter. That was her heart and soul, too.

She's gonna be just fine.

Brock

I met Brock for the first time when he was five or six. He was riding his bike in circles around this cul-de-sac. He barely noticed me. We moved in together around his ninth birthday. This was after a "courtship" that felt shorter than a one-night stand. So here's me and this kid, near strangers, just hanging out under one roof.

So, hey, I'm your stepmom.

Hey, great.

Okay.

I always wanted to marry a guy with a kid. I figured it would take the pressure off. "The mother instinct" hadn't kick in. I was thirty-four. I'm guessing it should've kicked in by then. So, the best thing to do was to find a nice guy who already had a kid with *another* woman, that way there'd be no pressure for me to reproduce. Mission accomplished. I wanted them to be older, too. Not in the mood to deal with the toddlers. Mission doubly accomplished. And I was really hoping that "them" would be a "him." He'd have Dad, and my role as stepmom would be even further diminished seeing as how we were not of the same sex. It was like I hit the trifecta.

Little did I know. I hit the jackpot with Brock. First of all, this kid was so tall that nine looked more like twelve on him, and he was treated as such. I'm guessing I wasn't the first person in his life that expected more out of him solely because we were nearly eye-level. I'm not saying this kid doesn't have faults, but he came into my life with two great parents who've taught him well. Brock and I have been able to form an atypical stepmom to stepson bond: we're friends. When he's in the mood to ramble, I'm here to answer all the questions he's not in the mood to ask his parents. He digs that I lived in L.A. We talk about that a lot. He has a very laid-back personality, whereas I'm very extreme. He's so mellow that his energy actually adds a nice calming effect to a pretty rattled household.

When Gram moved in, Jazz lost her room. We had to stash every pink thing she owned into Brock's. For months, their things stayed mingled and piled on top of each other. He didn't say a word.

Gram wasn't very warm or welcoming with him. Her disease had progressed just enough to permanently shut the door on "new" faces. She'd been around him a bit, but not steadily enough to believe he was family. He's never said a word about it.

She never knew his name. That just got silly. We must have called him "Bart" for six months after one of her greetings. He'd smile knowingly without complaint.

She couldn't deal with him eating. He's almost fifteen and stands over six-five. The kid needs to eat. But according to Gram, all food in fridge is stamped "Property of Jazz." Still, Brock just grabs his plate, bares a mischievous smile, sneaks away, and doesn't say a thing.

A few times Pete and I really needed a break. It'd be a Friday or Saturday night, and we just wanted one beer and a little conversation outside these four walls. Brock would stay with Gram. He didn't argue or whine. He didn't say a word.

She'd snarl about whatever. He'd slide past her and nod. She'd talk about him as though he weren't in the room. He'd just stand behind her with a grin and shrug.

We turned his world on its side. Nora Jo wasn't *his* grandma. He had no attachment to her. She has a mental illness and blew in like a tornado into his breeze-free adolescent existence. The needs of the house were dramatically and suddenly altered. To a kid his age, that could have been disastrous. He's seen her lost, confused, angry, drunk, injured, sick, tormented, sad beyond belief, and probably even naked. But I wouldn't know about it. He's held strong to his impeccable manners. He's made a few comments in jest, nothing malicious, just pretty funny. And when things have gotten really crazy, he'd come to me on the D.L. (down-low), no attitude in sight. It's like when it comes to my gram he's never heard of the word complain. He "gets" it. Damn, it'd be great to be half that cool.

Pete

"This really is bullshit. This whole thing with Nor. Lis says I'm closed off. I need to "emote." That's her term, not mine. Our marriage has been really put to the test since all this started, and I guess I'm supposed to talk about it. But doesn't that defy who I am? This closed off dude. And then she throws in some crap about me being a Scorpio ... and it's all so gay that I have to tap the volume up a notch on ESPN just to get through the harassment. My parents were divorced by the time I was two and I grew up with three older sisters nagging my ass like sisters are supposed to do. I've lived through some shit, like the Gulf War. And I've done my share of living, too. And a lot of those roads have led to women—and they keep leading to women. *That much is clear to me now*. I guess what I'm saying is, "I bit the bullet." And not just by getting married. If you've read up to this point, look who I married? Not exactly your average, sweet-talking, soft-speaking, submissive cup of tea. Some days, she's more like the drug you choke down to take the edge off the worst hangover of your life only to discover it escalates it—*to the point of puking*. Other times, it's like I'm living with three more women—wait a minute—that part's true. There's Lis, Jazz, and her mom, and then we switched out Sherie for Nor. And that's when I lost my bedroom to a high-energy three-year-old who's a cover-stealer and big-time wiggler. Lis has put some sort of feng shui all over the house that's supposed to create harmony. Did I just say feng shui? Seriously, look what these women have done to me! On the other hand, I'm beginning to think the house would have imploded by now if not for these crazy little crystals hanging from our ceilings. It's been a long cold winter. And Lis has had an extra harsh day with Nor. She's had a bunch thanks to an unforgiving string of bitter-cold months."

"So, how was your day?" I uttered tentatively, unsure of her mood which has been known to fluctuate wildly minute to minute. (It used to be day to day, now it changes by the minute.)

"Great. Just great. Let's see ... it involved threats, vulgarity, bodily excrement, alcohol, pubic hair, prescription drugs, and eventual brainwashing."

"Sounds like every day in middle school."

God, she looked tired, but I saw her raise an eyebrow. Oh—I made her laugh. This is good, this is good.

"I go to school everyday with this special ed degree in my back pocket in the hopes of changing just one kid's life. That's at 7:30 in the morning. I leave at 3:30 hoping no one winds up in jail by sundown. *Go to college. Get your ass into the Armed Forces. Just don't go to prison. And graduate from high school.* Please, at the very least, get your high school diploma. That was my dad's hope for me—to graduate from high school and stay out of jail. I went way beyond those expectations. On days when my wife is 'out of her head,' I wish I hadn't shot so high. But here I am living with Sybil, Mother Teresa, and Janeane Garofalo all rolled into one. And that's just Lis! Nor? I love Nor. She's a simple woman who took care of her family all her life and she deserves that much in return. And comforting Nor comes easy. She needs an ear, a hug, and a beer—always in that order. So finally, I can put a number on the lives outside of my kids that I know I'm truly impacting. That number is one. Nora Jo. Yeah, our lives feel like a series of blows with just enough space in between to let you catch your breath. And the marriage is either in melt-down or recovery mode. But it's no one's fault. It is what it is. Hey, if you're expecting me to go deeper, I can't. I'm closed off. *Remember?* But it's cool. I'm happy I got it in me to be there for Lisa's Gram, even though eventually she'll have no recollection of it. Right now, in Nor's eyes, I'm 'the man of the house.' She comes from the generation where men are 'key.' My presence in this home puts her at ease. But there will come a day when I will go from the man who's made her dinner and locks the doors at night to a stranger who's helping her on with her coat to an obsolete structure who's every move is foreign and frightening. The one person whose life I have willingly, positively, and with heartfelt sincerity made an impression on, won't remember any of it. She won't know my name. She won't know my gender. She'll forget how to walk and she'll forget how to talk. So why would she remember me? Theoretically, I get it. But I don't know if it'll stop me from thinking: *Nor, It's me. I'm 'the man,' Pete. I'm that guy that cooks for you ... you gotta know that much? We've laughed, we've drank, we've danced. I've saved you from a couple of falls and picked you up after a few, too. I'm the guy that gives you such good hugs. It's me, Pete.* But none of that will mean anything to her. And that's the part that really is bullshit."

Chapter Ten

"Step out of your reality and into theirs."

Laura Bramley
Author of *Elder Care Read*

A Million Miles Away

ete asked me the cautious question, "Have you thought about whether it's time?"

I have.

My personal goal has been surpassed. She has been with us for well over a year. The future inevitably became the present and I am faced with the same nagging question. Except now, the deterioration of her mind is moving at a steady, impressive pace.

"Have you thought about whether it's time?" He questioned carefully again. Apparently I didn't answer the first time. I'm all caught up in my third beer and "Breaking Dawn," the fourth and final of "The Twilight Series." Can you blame me for not answering?

I heard him. Was thinking about it. But had no answer. So I sat there like an idiot, sipping my Killian's. Finally, my shoulders twisted into a lame-ass shrug. "Yeah." That seemed to momentarily placate him (even though I'm pretty sure he just took that as a "no").

Welcome to one of those strange backward moments when "yes" actually means "no." Welcome to our lives.

How can I put this woman in a nursing home? I keep ensuring people that she still has her "faculties" and when that finally goes—when I'm cleaning up shit and piss from her sheets and from my grandfather's BVDs, then it'll be time.

Then I move on to my next inner squabble. The wannabe lawyer in me has been known to "counterpoint" all over the place. *I'll wait for now, but definitely move her into a home when she no longer knows who I am. That way she won't be sad. There. Challenge that you So-n-So's.*

For the last six months of my Grandpa Fritz's life, he uttered few phrases beyond "That's a jim-dandy, boy!" and "You betcha, Charlie!" And he did this with a permanently painted grin while rubbing that tabletop in constant clockwise circles. It bothered no one and kept him at ease. Yet, two weeks before he died, I came in as I did daily, greeted him with a kiss (another daily occurrence) and then he greeted me with a surprising, "Hello, Lisa. How are you?"

Ten days later, he was in a home. You see, "he" had lost control of his faculties. What was anyone to do? What was Gram to do? Nobody had a choice.

He lived four more days.

The day before he died, God graced me with the gift of cutting his hair. My dad had me cutting hair since I was twelve. One day he handed me a pair of scissors and said, "Cut my hair." Dad never asked so much as ordered. As a result, I'm the family "hair cutter."

So I had the pleasure of cutting my grandfather's hair one last time. Upon finishing, he gazed up and said, "Thank you." Then he touched my arm. His eyes were filled with tears (something I had never seen) when he uttered, "Please come back and see me tomorrow."

"I promise, Gramps. I promise. I will be here tomorrow." I put my hand over his, choked on my own tears and looked intensely into his loving eyes until it seemed certain that he believed me. Then we slowly let go of each other and I walked down that sterile hallway toward the exit, leaving him with half-living strangers gathered about the halls in wheelchairs and walkers, looking at nothing, thinking about less.

He died late that night in his sleep.

Pete told me the next day. My mom didn't want to wake me in the wee hours of morning. A panicked cry shuddered from my body rhythmic and jittery, but was quickly calmed by the logical notion that his journey was finally over. He was free and at peace. And most importantly, with his son—my dad.

I would have visited that next day as promised, but was secretly grateful that it was no longer possible.

This woman in my house, Nora Josephine Cerasoli, has been like a mother to me (and I already have a pretty phenomenal mother). I'm the girl who's been lucky enough to have two. How many people can say that? This woman in my home would have gladly given her life for me at any point, including now. That's why she fell so hard in the kitchen with Jazz. She was ensuring that "the baby" stay safe at all costs. Her entire existence has been one of "servitude." And she's never had the prefix "self" before it—not when she was a girl, and not as a woman, mother, grandmother, or wife.

She hates being alone. Her generation never knew about "Me" time, so it's not really her fault. And she hates being alive, too, most days. But that is a newer discovery. The woman buried behind disease, grief, and confusion never had anything but love to offer and, just like her cheese ravs, there were endless, generous portions of it.

I am stifled by constant thoughts. They're like reruns, the ones you're sick of seeing. I live in-the-now, like all the books tell me to, but it ain't easy because my "now" means waiting. My "now" means getting through another relentless, redundant day with Gram. My "now" means explaining for the hundredth time that Jazz is my daughter. She is her great grandmother. Pete is my husband. Brock is his son. Sherie is my mom. This is our house. Her room is the one at the end of the hallway in the lovely shade of hospital green. She has lived here for a year and a half. We have sold her house. Two very nice young people live there with their small children. The money is in the bank. She has beer in the laundry room sink where she's always kept it. It's Tuesday. It's Wednesday. It's morning. It's night. It's January. It's June. It's 2009. You are eighty-eight. We're not going to have a hurricane— that was national news. Jazz is my daughter. Pete is my husband. Sherie is my mother ...

It's been so exhausting.

I used to love her, oh, yeah, but I had to kill her.

I used to love her, oh, yeah, but I had to kill her.

I had to put her, six feet under.
She's buried right in my backyard...
And I am so going to Hell.

"Step out of your reality and into theirs." That's what Laura Bramley recommends in her book, *Elder Care Read.* So that's my new mantra. And I've worked daily to incorporate this simple suggestion into the way in which Gram is cared for. Some days it works and my head hits the pillow guilt-free. Lucky me. Most days it's a struggle. I want to scream every memory, however unfortunate they may be, because the woman she used to be is sorely missed. I want her to remember that Dickie was my dad— *her son*, and she was a great cook, and she always had a smile on her face, and loved going for walks, and gardening ... *and she was even into dogs.*

It's important (to me) that she knows that not only did my dad exist, but he's the guy that died young and of cancer, not Gramps. My grandfather "fell asleep" at the ripe old age of eighty-seven. She mourns the loss of Fritz, but never my father, and that's really bothersome, especially to my mother. My mother bites her tongue every time Gram talks about "her Fritz."

It's because deep down she can't deal with the loss of my dad. We both know that. Dementia has locked his memory someplace safe, someplace far from instant consciousness, sort of like a self-preservation technique. Is this the one small gift this cunning illness has to offer? Or did pain of this magnitude—the pain of losing a child—aid in the onset of the disease in the first place? Honestly, I'll never know. But never hearing her speak my dad's name or mourn his loss like she does grandpa's bothers me, too, though neither of us will ever tell her that.

On days when she'd lock herself in the bathroom because she needed a shower because it's been weeks and she's been dodging me and she smells like ... well ... like *it's been weeks*—those are the days the urge to scream stalks me.

"Just leave me alone. Leave me in here to die! Take me to a home! I don't need anyone! Leave me in here to die, goddamnit!" Her words permeate through the solid oak door.

This went on for hours one time in particular.

I tried begging.

Bitching.

I called Pete at school four times for advice.

Finally, Jazz, my genius, suggested we write G.G. a note. Then she dashed with glorious energy for marker and paper before I even had a chance to respond.

The note read:

I love you G.G.,

JAZZ

The entire blurb was straight from the splendid brain of my remarkable four-year-old.

She slipped it excitedly under the door like she just discovered the cure for cancer and was breaking the news to the rest of the world.

A moment passed.

The door finally swung open.

My future scientist, brain surgeon, president, astronaut, new millennium Picasso was beaming brilliantly despite the fact that staring back at us was an angry, naked, dripping wet old lady who's been sponge bathing herself for the last four hours. I watched as her face grew slowly sedated from the tiny "love note" clutched in her wrinkled, bruised, fragile hand.

I calmed down, too, and incorporated a soothing, cool edge to my voice (actually, that's a lie—I was just spent). "It's foolish to be mad at me for wanting to shower you, Gram. Do you see how foolish that is? We just want you to be clean. Jazz and I are here to take care of you. Please don't be mad at us for trying to do that. It's our job."

"It's our job, G.G." Jazz leapt, bare butt and all, into the bathroom and wrapped her arms tight around one of Gram's pasty, spider-veined legs. Then she added, "And please don't stay in the bathroom till you die 'cause we love you!"

I stared at these two incredible creatures wondering where and when life took such an extreme turn for the weird ... and somehow wonderful. One of them is too young to have developed any issues about the human body, the other has simply forgotten where the boundaries of "appropriateness" lie. And there they stood, a near century apart, enveloped by the pure love they hold for each other. Honestly, after hours of door pounding, yelling, and a whole bunch of silent inner rage, this right here, this bizarre picture of Jazz and my Gram made it all worth it. Thank God I was "awake" when this precious moment struck. Seriously, *Thank you, God.*

As if to photograph it, I took a step back, then inhaled and permanently imprinted this sweet snippet sent from Above into my memory banks. Both Jazz and Gram lived in a place that's barely recognizable to all us regular people. They were both free. Authentic.

Wow.

Before envy seeped through all my veins, rationale swam in like a shot of adrenaline and catapulted me into the bathroom. I had to take care of the task at hand before this very rare mood was permanently altered.

Moments like those will be forever logged, but they don't decrease my desire to come up with a scheme that'll keep her hanging on. Maybe I could blurt fact upon fact into a tape recorder and keep it on constant playback? Or I could scribble her life's story all over the walls in her room, or tattoo it on her forearms?

Doesn't she want to hold onto who she is? How can she not control this? And why, above all, does she not seem to care? Does she think the sum of all that she is can be narrowed down to one dead son and *a little gold coin?* Is that why she's so free to forget and accept? Why is she so comfortable letting every memory slip away? Why can't she choose which ones of them should stay?

I am plagued, too, by this same disease that won't release her. She may be its official captive, but I'm left standing outside its stone cold prison walls which are too high to scale, too thick to penetrate, and too dense to hear beyond. I am powerless compared to dementia. Useless against this monster. As a result, my alcohol consumption has elevated to help numb the debilitating feelings of anger, loneliness, lethargy ... and uselessness. Then I pause to notice beyond my own cloud of selfish, self-induced smog that my grandmother's behavior has been bordering unerringly on that of my own. Our energies are commingling into something new and unusual that goes way beyond bathrobes, boot slippers, and a few coiled strands of DNA. We don't return phone calls. We can't be bothered with food unless absolutely necessary (or of the liquid kind). Sometimes it's "pajamas all day!" Other days we sit zoning out to the TV with nothing to say. We nod back and forth politely, just because.

Without Jazz, I'm not sure either one of us would get out of bed. Does she feel her crucial role in all this? Does my four-year-old know that she, too, can't seem to shed that extra Christmas weight? Does she know she carries the burden as well, even if by default?

Gram and I are somehow driving each other into a world we didn't know existed. We're both quite aware the trip will take us to some dark, merciless place. That much is clear. And this one-way trip is on a deserted, never-ending stretch of road that's free of stoplights and there's no sign of rain, nothing to slow us down in sight. Plus, our mode of transport seems to be equipped with an endless supply of fumes and moving pretty steady now.

Yet again, here we were. Waiting.

The shower went swimmingly. She dressed while I gathered hair gel, rollers, and her pink plastic hairpins. Then she cautiously made her way into the kitchen and sat in the chair I'd pulled next to the counter.

"Shit, it's only 1:70? Is it too early for a beer?" she asked, staring at the stove before smiling up at me, hopeful.

"I just turned the oven on, Gram. It's after four."

I cracked her one and poured it into a mug.

"Where's the baby?"

"She's in her room playing."

"Oh," she said, sipping her beer.

"Are you her mommy?"

"Yes, Gram, I'm her mommy," I said twirling a strip of her auburn-dyed hair about a roller. Then she held up a pink plastic hair pin. I snatched it and slid it in place. "Jazz is my daughter and you're her great grandmother. Isn't that great?"

"I love her to pieces. Now who is her daddy?"

"Pete is her daddy. He's my husband."

"Are you married, sweetheart? Well, hit me with a brick, I did not know that."

Now there's a thought.

"Sure you do, Gram. You were at the wedding. Pete's the guy that's always cooking for us."

She thought about this, then handed me another pink plastic pin and sipped more beer.

"Am I your mama then?"

"No, Gram. You are my grandma."

"I thought I was that baby's mama. You know I just love her to pieces."

"We all do, Gram."

"Are you married, sweetheart?"

"Pete is my husband. We are Jazzy's parents. Brock is his son. And Sherie is my mom."

"Sherie? Oh, Sherie. She's not my age?"

"No Gram, she's your daughter-in-law." And there it was. I'd screwed up and said it.

A strange sad look overcame her face.

"She was married to my Dickie."

I sighed so heavy it hurt. "Yes, Gram, yes. She was married to Dickie."

Tears welled instantly in her tired, tired eyes.

"Dickie. My son? Dickie was my son."

"Yes, Gram, yes. He was your son."

"He died so young. Oh, my Dickie." She wiped away a defiant, traveling tear.

"Yes, Gram, yes. I miss him, too."

I finished twisting the final roller into her hair, pinned it in place and put down the comb. Then I did something strikingly out of character—a task I had rudely handed over to Jazz months ago. I hugged my gram and held on tight.

Finally, we released. She told me she loved me, smiled big, held my face with both hands, and kissed me square on the lips—a move I've grown to expect since birth. But then her heavy, lost eyes roamed back into the depths of her diminishing mind, slowly becoming preoccupied with all my abrasive "truths," trying to separate them from all these different ones that she believes now to be her own.

Her head tilted, her eyes lost all focus. A glaze dripped over them like icing over the edge of a freshly baked cake. And she was lost again. Freed. Maybe she was searching for her seven-year-old boy. She might be wracking her brain for her ravioli recipe, or a clear glimpse of Fritz's face. In any case, it was no longer about my dad.

Exactly what she was contemplating, no one will ever know.

I took a step back and said a small prayer (which probably came out more like a grievance), then pressed my right hand to my chest, shoving the anxiety back down into my stomach.

It was that time again to do the only thing I knew how. I grabbed a Killian's for myself and stood where she could see me, in case my services would be needed. She fidgeted, mainly with that coffee mug. She took a hearty gulp, then patted the rollers in her hair, pleased with my work. The stove beeped, but it didn't seem to distract her. It was clear, at least for that moment, that I wouldn't be needed to drudge through another string of unresolved questions. So I tossed in the pizza, grabbed my beer from the counter along with my book, and curled up on the couch. It was hard cover, the novel, so peering over the top of it to study Gram was a cinch. There I was, pretending to read, but caught up in something sadly more intriguing, something that has perpetually taken me out of my "day." I was watching my grandmother, Nora Jo, as she slowly fades away.

Epilogue

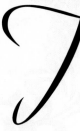 take out a thick, blue magic marker and a neon green 8x11 piece of card stock. More neatly than usual, I write:

> **Gram,**
> **Your child is NOT lost.**
> **He is with me.**
> **Go back to bed now.**
> **I love you,**
> **Lisa**

Then I find a thick roll of clear tape and affix this letter-sized note to her bedroom door at eye-level. I read it several times for spelling errors and clarity. I read it as if I were Gram. Then I read it one last time just because I'm a glutton for punishment.

This note doesn't provide quite the same entertainment as the one we adhered well over a year ago onto the microwave. My stomach churns like clockwork. I walk away hoping another obstacle has been briefly diverted. And it hits me: I no longer ponder over the goal that was surpassed since moving her in nearly two years back, or spend my days considering other options. Thoughts such as those have vacated my mind. It's moment to moment with Gram now. So I hurdle the episodes and oddities that this illness brings on like I'm Prancer herself, and then seize the breaks that grace us during the uneventful in-betweens. It's me vs. dementia, and I'll be damned if my dukes aren't up, in position and waiting for word from the king. It's no longer about "when." It's about "how." How can we all survive today? Letting go of the goal has alleviated some of the tension at Chez Weaver. That's the good news.

But the thing about dementia or Alzheimer's (whatever the label) is the "funny" fades as the need for care increases. So, as you work harder and harder and harder—to the point of severe fatigue and near insanity—your job grows increasingly less rewarding. The result at the end of this trial is not a promotion, a degree, a huge Christmas bonus, or even a little "congrats" followed up by a pat on the back. It's death. Your "job" ends when your "caseload" dies. And all your efforts are to be rewarded to you not here, not now, but later in Heaven. *Isn't that awesome?* I guess it is, if you believe you're going to Heaven. Or if you believe in Heaven at all anymore after what you and your family have witnessed and endured.

I'm tossing and turning par course, when I finally whisper to

Pete over our sleeping little girl, "You know, after spending the better part of a year caring for my dad, I thought, finally, the one real thing that would get me into Heaven was finally behind me. I didn't ask for it, didn't want it, but surprised myself and pulled it off."

"I know you did, babe." he whispers back and squeezes my hand.

"And then Gram comes along and I figure, okay, apparently God thinks 'someone' needs to do a little more. Or maybe it's karma. I'm paying off some more karma."

"Yeah. I know the feeling, babe."

"And I thought, no problem, God. I got this one."

"Yeah, I know you did."

But I don't "got this one."

He squeezes my hand one more time and tickles my palm with his fingertips. That was sign language for, "But you will. You're figuring this out. Give yourself a break."

To get tragically personal, I'll confess that at no point when I was taking care of my dad did the urge to punch him ever enter my consciousness. I'm guessing the impulse to punch cancer patients rarely comes up. *But dementia?*

I am most positive that this on-again/off-again desire to physically beat the dementia right out of Gram has and will remain just that—a harmless urge. But it's nothing to be proud of. I've lost my temper, had to leave the room and sometimes the house. A couple of times, I've actually left the state and got my mother or some other capable but otherwise clueless innocent to cover.

This experience has been challenging on a level only God

knows—well, Him and Pete. Am I doing the best job? I'm slowly getting better at the task before me. As gram gets harder to manage, I am surprisingly improving as a caregiver. I'm doing my personal best because that's who I am. It just doesn't feel like enough. I'm ill equipped, faking my way through this like the audition I didn't have time to prepare for. I'm a professional, so putting on a pretty good show and receiving rave reviews from friends has been easy. But at the end of the day when tired and tortured ring in as themes, it doesn't feel like success. And my prayers? Underneath your basic "standards" these contrary wishes sneak in asking Him to make it all end.

Care giving is a team sport. That's my latest revelation. When I could no longer look in the mirror at a smile-less face that's guilty of misplaced anger and cruel contemplations, that's when I discovered this angle to the game. So I set myself temporarily free now and again. We get a Grandma sitter. And Pete's discovered to his surprise and dismay that I still do enjoy the simple things in life like food and sex and conversations that aren't always about bodily functions, dead relatives, and long lost children.

And right now we like each other again. Most days.

I'd like to establish some kind of regular assistance, and a workout partner, a drinking buddy (a less repetitive drinking buddy), or even a praying buddy so at least a few hours a week I can feel like ME for a spell. A vacation is good, but some consistency might be wonderful. Maybe it would save the both of us—Gram from seeing only the overworked granddaughter who's losing her pace, and me from going to Hell for not doing a better job. Maybe regular mini-breaks will make me want to break out my figure-flattering jeans again. Maybe they'll remove the feeling of being captured and caged. Or stop me from thinking, woe is me or *what am I doing? Or...*

What was I thinking in the first place?

I look up from my computer as Nora Jo shuffles toward the window. She sits cautiously on the bar seat. It's high for her, so she's extra careful. A cup of coffee is already on the table in front of her. It's one of three wandering mugs she's made so far today. She takes a satisfied sip, clarifying that this one is the freshest. I'm at the edge of her periphery, yet she doesn't see me. And I'm quiet, too, on purpose. I want to blend in with the rest of the fixtures, the curtains, the plants, the table—and go unnoticed.

She seems sad.

Suddenly her gaze slowly shifts from melancholy to a complete blankness. A pile of abysmal tears gather swiftly inside my eyes. I can't move, but wonder if she can hear my heart beating right out of my chest from halfway across the room. I circle it a couple of times habitually. *Come on Panic, get back in there.* The moment I've feared has arrived. I'm strangled silent by its presence.

Minutes pass …

I picture her looking over and asking me my name. Or turning and screaming at the sheer shock of my foreign presence. Or maybe her eyes wander over and she wants to scream at the sight of me, but nothing comes out because she can't remember how. And then I imagine she's catatonic. She won't turn at all. And I will study her lonely, crooked, willowy figure staring blankly into a world that no longer holds any meaning whatsoever. Then I'll have to be the one to get up, go over, and finally face this enemy who's been creeping in corners and shadows among us for so long.

Maybe I should call my mom? 911 has got nothing on Mom. That's what I'll do. As soon the rhythm of my breath steadies and this force field that's rendered me motionless lifts, I'll call my mom. In the meantime, I wish I could take back every wicked little prayer that willed this finale into my life. You see, I'm just not ready yet.

Suddenly, like a drowning person ejects a gulpful of water and life rushes back into their skin, Gram's face expels the void that was holding it hostage ... *and she's back.*

She tilts her head in my direction and smiles. For her, no time has passed.

I raise a hand and wave. And for the first time in this journey, I am out of my head and at peace in my plight.

I've lost many freedoms,
But still have my mind.
I can't go to a movie on a whim,
And can no longer work full-time.

A good night's sleep is a thing of the past.
And my short-term memory is for shit,
I lose my cell phone twice as often,
And exercise without breaking a sweat.

My husband and I have lost our bedroom,
Jazz has become a permanent figure.
Most days are welded together and heavy.
I no longer wake up to tomorrow eager.

I've lost many freedoms,
But still have my mind.
As for my gram?
It's a race against Time.

She's lost her two kitchens.
That must be Hell for a cook.
She wanders aimlessly in her "new" home,
No safe place to look.

She, too, can no longer sleep.
Her nights are mixed up with her days.
And years' past swoop down to strangle her,
Her reality? An inescapable maze.

Gram lost her husband five years ago,
Her bed is lonely and so cold.
After a lifetime of companionship,
The covers "to her left" lack reason to fold.

She lives without a purpose,
And works hard to break into smile.
Uselessness precedes her every move,
And getting out of bed takes more than "a while."

I've lost many freedoms,
But still have my mind.
But my gram is losing everything,
And all at the same time.

It hardly seems fair to me,
That a woman who is so beautiful,
Didn't end up with a better angel,
To protect her from this private Hell.

I'm no saint and I'm no savior,
And I can't raise a dead son from his grave.
All I really got is this idea
That she's my family to support and save.

And this plan I have has failed before,
And I'm certain this is no new show,
But I know my spirit will prevail,
For it came from a place called "Nora Jo."

The Photo Album

Nora Josephine McMahon
Born March 18, 1921
Approximate age in photo is sixteen

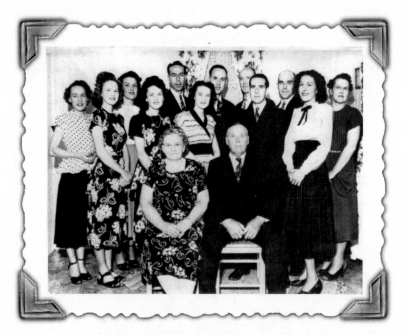

The McMahon Family early 1930s
Seated: Parents John and Mary
Left to right front row: Aggie, Ila, Ruthie, Billy, Nora
Back row: Vern, Irella, George, Pat, Harold, Ralph, Helen

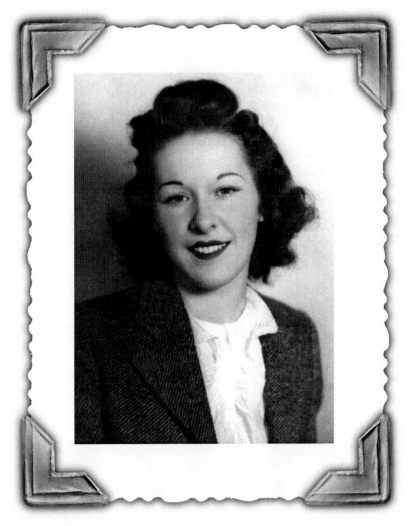

Nora Josephine Cerasoli

Mid-1930s

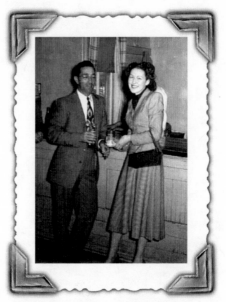

Fritz and Nora mid-1940s

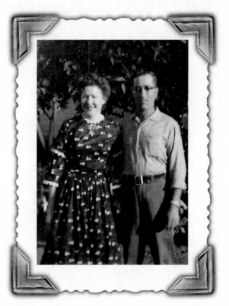

1962
Iron Mountain, Michigan

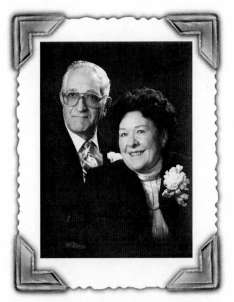

50th Wedding Anniversary
May 4, 1988

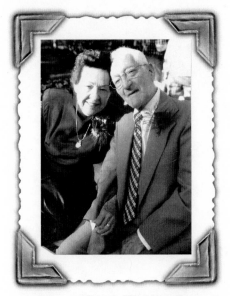

Pete and Lisa's Wedding Day
September 20, 2003

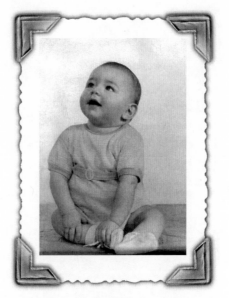

Richard "Dickie" Cerasoli
Born: July 5, 1943

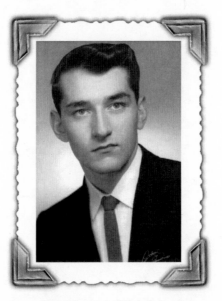

Iron Mountain High School
Graduation Photo, 1961

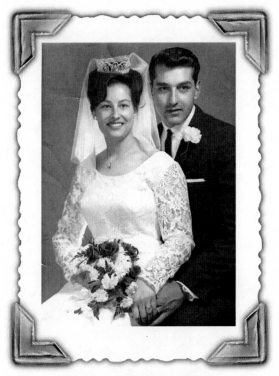

Charlene "Sherie" DeMeuse
Richard "Dick" Cerasoli
May 29, 1965

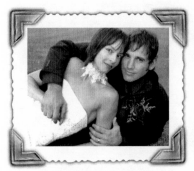

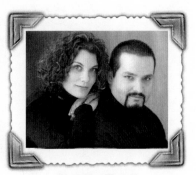

Lisa Marie Cerasoli
Raymond Peter Weaver
September 20, 2003

Jennifer Tyrell
Richard Alfred Cerasoli
December 27, 2005

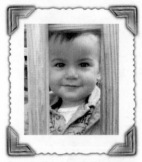

Jacob Richard Cerasoli
Born: March 9, 2008

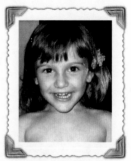

Jazzlyn Jo Weaver
Born: June 1, 2005

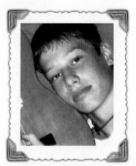

Brock Lewis Weaver
Born: September 29, 1994

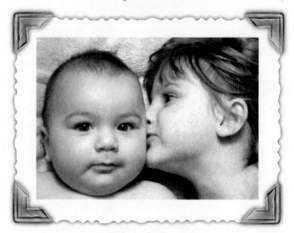

Jakey & Jazz
Summer 2008

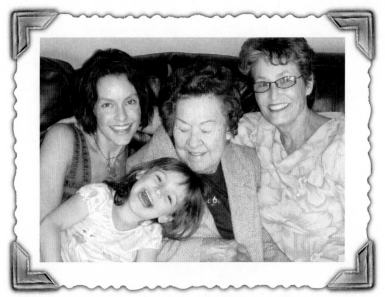

Lisa, Jazzy Jo, Nora Jo and Sherie Cerasoli
Four Generations of Silly Ladies
Mother's Day 2009

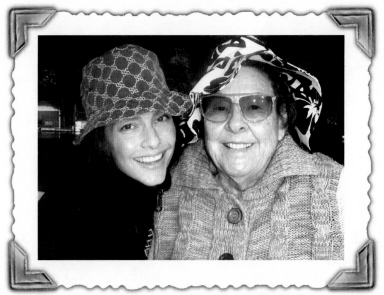

Lisa and Gram on "The Chain of Lakes"
Spread Eagle, Wisconsin 2009

In Memory of...

This project, like so many other things, has opened yet another
door in my life, proving once again just how connected
we all are here on planet Earth.

The stories and poems on the following pages are a tribute to
the victims of dementia, Alzheimer's and other related illnesses
written by surviving loved ones.

They are thought-provoking, delightful, eloquent and heart
wrenching, too. And most of them have come from people
whom I have never met.

I'm honored they are a part of this memoir.

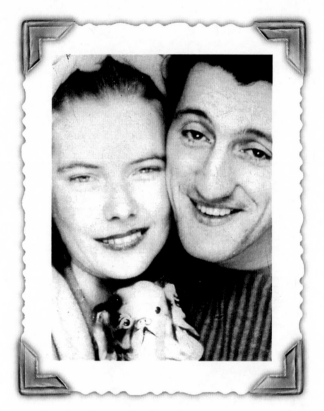

Marion Rhodes Calo
February 25, 1921 ~ August 8, 2005

Y MOTHER, MARION RHODES CALO was a woman of unparalleled inner and outer beauty. As a young child, she took on the unusual but necessary responsibility of caring for her three siblings. This experience is what made Marion a remarkably strong woman. As an adult, being a loving wife and mother brought Marion the true happiness of her existence. Family always came first!

I was with my mother when the doctor gave her a test to check her memory. He asked simple questions. *Do you know what day it is? Can you tell me what month we're in? Do you know who our current president is?* Her eyes grew wide with anxiety. She looked over at me with the hope I could help. Of course, I could not. It was so heart breaking to see her realize her disability. I watched helplessly as fear crept over her face.

It was not long after the day of her "diagnosis" that she began a nightly routine of kissing every picture of the family and saying their names out loud. Marion wasn't going to let Alzheimer's take her beloved family away from her. That was her one mission. She won that battle. Till her dying day, she never forgot who we were.

I look back at so many fond memories, but also recall some impatience I had with my mother. She liked to watch me put on my makeup everyday ... and it bugged me. I asked her frequently not to watch, stating it made me nervous. Now that she's gone, I'd give anything to have her sitting there watching me. It has been hard for me to deal with those misguided behaviors. Since I can no longer apologize, I've tried my best to remedy them. My vanity now boasts a beautiful, smiling picture of my mother. She gets to watch me everyday now. And she remains forever in my heart.

I love you, Mom!

Your Daughter,
Grace Calo Tullis
Novato, California

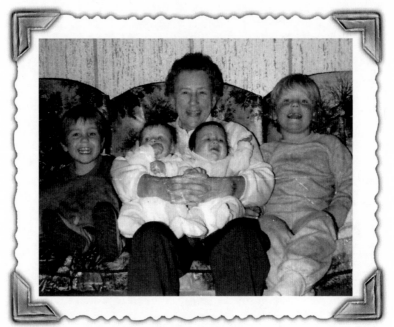

Evelyn Smith
January 29, 1913 ~ February 14, 2009

The Heart Remembers...

The mind remembers her blank stares to places that seemed afar, but the heart remembers her cookies in the gold and white cookie jar.

The mind remembers her wearing the same clothes day after day, but the heart remembers that beautiful red dress she wore on my wedding day.

The mind remembers going to the nursing home, wondering if she'd be well, but the heart remembers sitting on her porch, listening to the stories she'd tell.

*The mind remembers her looks of being lost and forlorn, but
the heart remembers the joy she felt when her grandchildren
were born.*

*The mind remembers the fuss she'd make looking for Daddy hour after
hour, but the heart remembers the magic she'd make with apples, sugar
and flour.*

*The mind remembers her seeming fragile and frail, but
the heart remembers her smiling while filling her blueberry pail.*

*The mind remembers her getting thin and that her clothes no longer fit,
but the heart remembers the beautiful afghans and baby sweaters she'd
knit.*

*The mind remembers leaving, her face branded with a hint of shame,
but the heart remembers the look you would get if you messed up the
Canasta game.*

*The mind's memories are a funny thing and with time, will lessen and
fade, but the heart's memories will last forever, for they were
Heaven made.*

Your Loving Granddaughter,
Diane M. Hecht
Leslie, Missouri

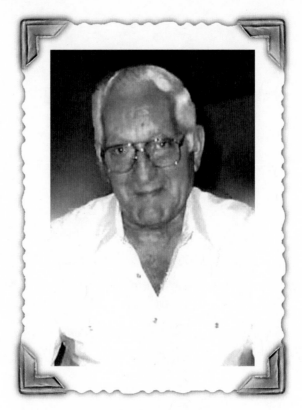

Alfred "Fritz" Cerasoli
August 23, 1916 ~ June 21, 2004

A Look and a Giggle

June 1980

I AM SIX YEARS OLD SITTING AT THE KITCHEN table with my grandpa Fritz. He puts his hand over mine, I put my other over his. He puts his other hand on top of our already stacked hands. I move my bottom hand to the top of his, and so on. We do this for hours—it was our game. Of course, the man always let me win. God, I loved him.

My grandfather was always so happy and accepting. I always felt so comfortable around him. I could be myself no matter what. Whatever turmoil was rolling within our family, he was a calming breeze in the storm. Gramps always had his patented giggle and a somewhat hidden but knowing smile. The man was not only my rock both physically and mentally, he was a secure place of refuge for everybody. Even as a child, I was in awe of that.

Gramps had a full white head of hair, was always clean shaven and had this glow on his face like he understood life in a way nobody else did. It was a look of pure happiness like he held the key to a secret room with an endless amount of joy and he frequented the place regularly. Since my grandfather's death, the joy that used to brighten up my day vanished in an instant, like so many small gifts in life you don't know you have until they are taken away.

August 2003

I am a twenty-nine-year-old man, or at least what I thought approximated a man. Boy, was I off. I am sitting next to my Grandfather on the couch choking back tears. I am a complete stranger to him. He is completely terrified, both of me and the surroundings. I slowly place my arm over his shoulders and gently reassure him, "It's okay, Gramps, I'm here." I do this knowing full well I no longer exist in his narrowing world.

Grandpa Fritz quickly gets up off the couch and starts

systematically searching for his son, Richard. My father had died four weeks prior, after spending nine months battling lung cancer. I corral him back to the couch and painfully explain that his baby boy had died at age sixty. The old comforting familiarity of his face crumbles and reflects confusion and deep unhappiness. This was one of the worst moments of my life—a moment which would be replayed several times throughout the day due to his deteriorating state of awareness from Alzheimer's.

This disease robbed my grandfather of his personality and of his memories. The man who existed three years before his death was now trapped within a body and world he didn't understand or recognize. And all this was happening while he was going deaf and blind. His once noteworthy and signature giggle—the one I knew so well—had now become a defense mechanism to mask fear and misplaced memories.

My family has learned the difficult way that Alzheimer's robs more than just from the individual suffering. It also raids family and friends of cherished time (even though love can in no way be diminished by any disease). It can also push loved ones and caregivers to the edge of insanity. But with faith and a strong hold on past memories, Love and Compassion will prevail.

You were the best, Gramps.

Love,
Richard "Alfred" Cerasoli
Detroit, Michigan

Eleanore Micke
June 25, 1917 ~ February 19, 2009

M Y HUSBAND RON AND I WENT TO my grandmother one day back in the spring of '07. We walked into her room in the Alzheimer's wing. There was my gram sitting in a chair by the window, looking lovely as ever. She was always a woman who took great pride in her appearance. She was elegant and perfectly poised, and today was no exception. Fortunately, she was still at a stage in the disease where she knew me, so we greeted each other warmly. Then she asked, "So, where are you living now?"

I hadn't moved in eighteen years. "I still live in Gladstone."

Grandma looked as if that made sense. She was onto her next question. "What are you doing there?"

"I stay at home with the kids."

She grew momentarily quiet, then proceeded to repeat those same two questions over and over, as-a-matter-of-factly. By the third or fourth round, I turned to Ron wondering how long this line of questioning was going to persist.

So where do you live?

And what are you doing there?

I smiled and repeated, "I stay at home with the kids."

She nodded and added, "Oh, so you sit on your ass all day."

My husband nearly fell off the bed.

As for me, it was the first time I heard my grandmother swear. I was shocked, but readily recovered, and am grateful for the memory. It brings a smile to my face every time.

With Love,
Jill Spencer
Gladstone, Michigan

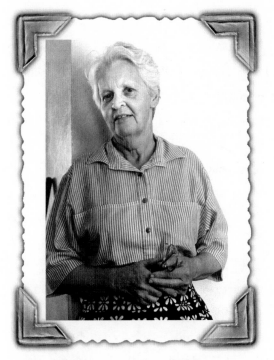

Joyce Provencher Gagnon
November 26, 1925 ~ October 26, 2006

*I*T'S BEEN THREE YEARS—THREE LONG YEARS without the amazing presence of my mother Joyce here on this ambivalent earth. Even in the throes of Alzheimer's disease for sixteen years, she molded lives in a spiritual, loving and positive way up to and beyond the time of her death.

Mingled we were in the end. With my head nestled in her chest, I listened longingly to the slowing of her heartbeat. This beautiful, unforgettable woman was wrapped in my arms when her last breath left her body. It was my last chance to absorb the essence of the best person I've ever known, and I seized it. Peace was finally delivered to the most deserving, most incomparable of Alzheimer's victims. An honor, a sacrifice, and a painful, yet treasured memory is how I've described that experience. It's indelibly marked in my heart and mind. And it happened on my son's twelfth birthday.

As a former nurse who contracted tuberculosis in the 1940s and survived it, she lived life under the Latin code of "Carpe Diem." She had ten children and toiled and nurtured ceaselessly to make life sweeter for everyone.

She was a lover of light: sunrise, sunset, the night sky, a full moon and campfires. She was also a true artist. I'd watch quietly as she'd mix oil paints timidly on a canvas. Then I'd amaze at how it slowly came to life, and we'd both delight at the new sensation she alone created. Her laugh was lilting and pure. Her songs, sung in a rich alto, comforted and delighted, and her fingers on the piano keys exuded joy.

She saw nature as the ultimate escape. She dressed down and rose up to meet the most challenging of elements—peeling pulpwood to make a needed dollar in sweltering July with flies the size of hummers buzzing around her head. She'd pile wood, pick rocks, and wake before dawn to fish, waiting to land morsels to feed the family, all the while enjoying the outdoors—her paradise. As a gardener, she tended to a four-lot expanse where she planted and grew every possible vegetable. She canned and froze and cooked her bounty and time stood still.

She held a baby, kissing a downy head, as if ... as if this baby in her arms was the most precious treasure of the universe. I had the honor of being one of those babies. She held me when my teeth were knocked loose from a skating accident. She set me straight when I was cocky. She saw the sincerity in my future husband's eyes. She traveled to the ends of the world with me on my first job interview. And when she battled tuberculosis, she wrote me letters from the sanitarium. I was two at the time. And she cradled me in her arms as we both wiped tears from each other's faces when my child, Camille, lost her battle to cancer at fourteen months old. She remembered the loss of her son, Rocke. And we both have shared the experience and concern of having a child with diabetes. And me? Even now at forty-nine I feel orphaned by her loss. I am lovely Joyce's bereft orphan.

Joyce's mother, Rita, was another victim of Alzheimer's—this insidious disease. And after a lifetime of love and dedication, my father died after witnessing the slow destruction and death of his "angel," my mother. He gave Joyce what she deserved—a life of happiness, comfort, security and care. And he became dust, tumbleweed, a tree without roots ... another victim of Alzheimer's. He died exactly a year to the day after her.

This forty-nine-year-old high-risk-for-Alzheimer's orphan pleads: Read this book. Learn about Alzheimer's. Support research to find a way to manage this inhumane monster. But mostly, I plead, as my mother and grandmother before me, and in honor of Nora Jo: "Carpe Diem." Seize the day.

In Loving Memory,
Wendy Zambon
Iron Mountain, Michigan

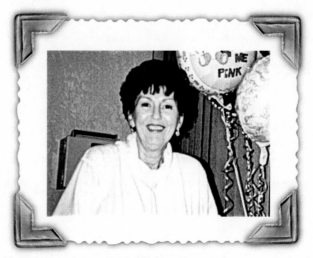

Jakie Pearce Pepper
May 6, 1936 ~ August 3, 2007

*M*Y MOTHER, JAKIE, WAS A VERY PROUD woman. She always had to look her best, even if that meant being late to every function she ever attended. When I was child, going out to eat was a bit of a chore. In fact, it was a three-hour production. That's how long it took my mother to get ready.

It had always bothered my mom how little I cared for my looks. In high school and college I had no desire to wear makeup or dress nicely. I owned a pair of sweats and a sweat jacket that I wore so often they had holes in them. One day, the set mysteriously disappeared. I cried over it. To this day, I'm sure my mother discreetly tossed them.

Although my mother loved me dearly, she often commented on my looks and hair. It was never quite the right style for her. Then she was diagnosed with Alzheimer's and she slowly stopped noticing how I looked or what I wore. And when my parents would visit me, we could finally go to dinner without my mother undergoing an unneeded, overextended makeover. I was amazed! This new mother wasn't so bad after all. I could get used to this, I thought. But in reality, I missed the old mom—the one who showed her love for me the only way she knew how—by helping me to look my best.

My mother's doctors were amazed with how well she continued to do her hair and makeup, way past the time that most Alzheimer's patients ceased to care about personal hygiene or appearance. I was convinced that it was so ingrained, it had turned into reflex. I also believed she would strive to "look her best" until that part of her memory was taken away.

One day, she got a little bit of the old spark back while applying makeup. I was watching her press lipstick to her lips with both perfect precision and joy, when suddenly she turned to me and said, "This is great stuff. You should try it sometime!" I had to laugh. She couldn't remember what the word for "lipstick" was, but by gosh she knew I needed it!

The irony in all this? I now wear makeup every day. Maybe as a reminder, maybe because she was right. But even more telling, my teenage daughter, Elizabeth wouldn't be caught dead without it. And she, just like my mother, Jakie, makes us late to every function. We've certainly come full circle.

Your Loving Daughter,
Betsy Pepper Grugin
Marquette, Michigan

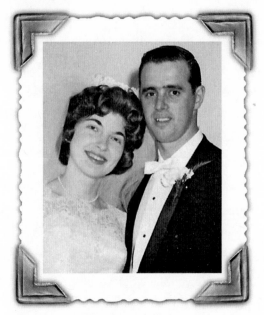

Donald Lee Siegler
October 27, 1939 ~ July 2, 2007

*W*HEN I TOOK THE VOW "FOR BETTER or worse, in sickness and in health," little did I know the true meaning of those words. But as life has gone on, the true meaning did indeed unfold.

I was married to Don, the love of my life, for forty-two years. We had a wonderful life. Don was a super husband, friend and the best father Larry and Janet could ever want. His life was dedicated to his children, and later his grandchildren. He was not only their father & grandfather, but their friend, coach and mentor.

Interest in sports has always been a Siegler family tradition. Shortly after our marriage, Don was given a set of golf clubs for Christmas. He mastered the game and also taught the children and me. We traveled the U.P. for many golf tournaments. Everyone wanted to know him and looked forward to seeing him each summer.

Don also spent a lot of time visiting his elderly mother who was in a nursing home with Alzheimer's. He was so compassionate. Little did he know he would be going down a similar path.

Oh how Don looked forward to retirement since he worked swing shift for most of his life. So at sixty-two he did it! Not long after that, he started having some problems with the recognition of certain "regular" objects. We took Don to a neurologist. At first they thought it was his medication, but as his condition got worse, they finally diagnosed him with "Picks" disease, a rare form of dementia which attacks the frontal temporal lobe of the brain… and starts with speech. By sixty-four Don had stopped talking altogether. That's when I realized that it's funny how after living with someone for forty years you know exactly what their needs are just by the look in their eyes. As his condition progressed, he remained the most wonderful patient, despite all the fear we were going through. Eventually he lost all ability to walk, and control of bodily functions including eating and swallowing.

With the help of a nurse, his loving children, and me, Don was able to stay in his own home. He was the youngest of four brothers, and they all helped, too, along with his sister, Nancy to ensure his life would be lived with dignity and in the place he wanted to be – HOME.

After five tough years, Don went to a better place. It was hard to let go, but he always reminded me that "we are just passing through."

As I reflect back over the past five years, it has been so comforting and given me so much peace knowing I was able to take care of Don. And I know he would have done the same for me.

He is sadly missed but most affectionately remembered.

His Beloved Wife,
Bernice Siegler
Norway, Michigan

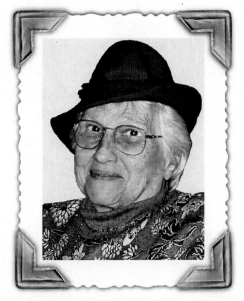

Pauline Cram
July 30, 1914 ~ November 3, 2009

"MA CRAM" IS HOW MOST PEOPLE referred to her. I called her "Gram, Gram Cram." Her given name was Pauline, though she was rarely called that, except by the priests she worked for. She created a life with my grandfather, Hiram and was always in service to others. They have nine surviving children who have had twenty-two grandchildren.

Ma Cram had an eighth-grade education along with the skills of a farmer's daughter in her tool belt, and used her faith as a blueprint to construct the big life she went on to lead. And lead she did. After my grandfather died at fifty due to diabetes complications, she chose to remain a widow and raise her family on her own.

The things that I remember most were the "smells" of Gram's home. Something sweet perfected in the oven while homemade noodles stretched over the backs of chairs. Her pots were like cauldrons as she cooked the only way she knew how to—for a crowd. She was the center of the universe, cooking in her home, and we were all glad to be in her orbit. She never missed a birthday and had family reunions on hers just to keep us close.

Gram was famous for her hats, her only vanity. They were in all shapes & colors from simple tams to a red felt hat with a scarlet plume. She was stunning in that one. I don't know what they meant to her, but there was a twinkle in her eye each time she wore one.

After the kids had all grown, she bought a large house and ran a foster care home for troubled teen girls. She became the house mother for a local fraternity. She cooked for the priests and nuns in her church and surrounding ones. She was devoted to her faith and would round up her wayward grandchildren each Sunday for Mass. This was before seatbelt laws, so she'd stack us all in like cord wood and then drive like a woman outrunning the devil himself on Big Bay Highway at speeds that kids fancied themselves "drag racing." She tapped her breaks only twice on that thirty mile strip, both spots had near ninety degree turns. And when she rounded them, an arm extended instinctively to protect her babies from the windshield. It was our "gram-go-go-gadget seatbelt."

She cared for me, my two older sisters and little brother, Pete, a great deal when we were younger. After bath time we got to have a treat and watch *The Lawrence Welk Show*. I think Gram had a crush on him. She'd sing along to "Tiny Bubbles" and swing us around while we giggled. She taught all the grandchildren to polka, sing, cook and pray. Pictures adorned her house of her family, Jesus and a picture of John F. Kennedy, her favorite president. Next to that was a framed copy of his famous speech, *"Ask not what your country can do for you…"* I remember reading this countless times as she sat detangling my hair after a bath. She thought he was so handsome, so did I.

Her body died on November 3, 2009, but Gram "left" before that. She had Alzheimer's. A series of strokes took away her ability to interact. I would go visit only if I had someone with me. I never got used to being an adult around Gram. And I mourned the passing of her spirit years before her body was laid to rest. Her funeral was a grand affair in contrast to her simple life. Over 500 people came for the showing, Mass and luncheon. All of the women in the family wore hats in her reverence. My uncle Joe, her youngest, drove the hearse back to Big Bay along the very highway she traveled daily. We reminded him to drive *all out* and only tap the brakes twice. Much to the distress of the funeral director in the passenger seat, he obeyed her "road rules."

My Gram spent her life filling ours with memories. It's a cruel irony that she was the first to forget them. But Alzheimer's cannot claim them from us. What is good, kind, fair and respectful in all her kin, is because of her influence. So thank you, Gram, Gram Cram.

Maggie (Weaver) Stang
Marquette, Michigan

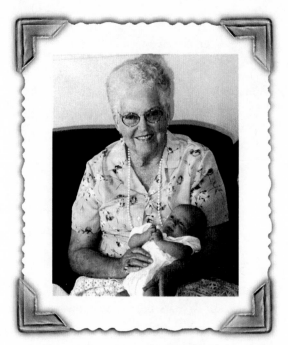

Allene Rowe Smith Nauta
March 27, 1925 ~ December 15, 2006

(A daughter and two granddaughters remember Allene.)

Seasons

Sharon Nauta Steele
Spanish Fork, Utah

Mama held me to her breast
And cooled my fevered brow,
Sang lullabies to help me sleep,
Shampooed my wispy, baby hair
And fed me with a spoon.

Heart to heart, we never guessed
years later, here and now,
I'd sing to her and pray and weep--
my mother, aging, in my care.
The years slipped by too soon.

With such a melancholy test,
I haven't figured how
to bridge this role reversal leap,
except, in knowing we share
mothering, commune.

Camping on the Desert
Jennifer Steele Christensen

NOT LONG AFTER WE WERE MARRIED and graduated from college, my husband Brad and I moved to Mesa, AZ, and we enjoyed the unique opportunity to visit Grandma & Grandpa in Quartzsite as they boon-docked on the desert. The only time I've ever eaten lobster was in their trailer one evening after we'd been to a huge flea market in town. Our "supper," as she always called it, was delicious, and I don't think the finest restaurant in the world could've topped it. It wouldn't have taken much, however, to top their shower. Because every drop of water is precious in the desert, Grandma & Grandpa had some amazing bathing system figured out. It seemed to me more like a spit shine, and I asked Grandma, "Are you sure this works?"

"Well," she answered, shrugging her shoulders, "Do we stink?"

I have to admit that I liked it best when Grandma & Grandpa visited us. I told them they could use all the water they'd like.

Don't Forget Me, Grandma!
Jennifer Steele Christensen

GRANDMA WAS VERY AFRAID OF LOSING her memory, and she used to make lists of things—people's names, landmarks, special events—to help her remember. Once, not long before she had to go to the nursing home, I took three of my children, Ammon, Camille, and Benjamin Rowe, who possesses her namesake, over to the house to visit. I was wearing a ball cap and had my hair pulled back in a pony tail. For just a moment, Grandma didn't recognize me. I took off the hat, let my hair down and said, "Look, Grandma, it's me, Jennifer!"

A few moments later, Ammon walked quietly over to Grandma and whispered, "Grandma, are you going to forget me?"

"No," Grams assured him, "You're my Ammon. Grandma will never forget you. I promise."

I want Ammon to know that Grandma kept her promise. Even though her memory failed her during her last years on earth, she kept us all in her heart. Where she is now, she knows us all, and God has given her back everything she lost, plus more.

Crocheting with Grandma
Monica Nauta Hanni

WHEN THINKING OF MY GRANDMA Nauta and the way she touched my life, many expressions of love come to my mind. Grandma was a wonderfully crafty woman. I remember her teaching me how to crochet. We started with a chain, and each time I would visit she would teach me a little more. Over the years, I lost most of it, but to this day I have never forgotten how to make a chain.

One of my fondest memories was at Christmas time when Grandma placed several tiny dolls on her tree. Each had a hand crocheted outfit and baby blanket in pink, yellow, and blue. On Christmas Eve, she sent each of her granddaughters home with one of those beautiful dolls.

I remember camping trips, parties, kind words, encouragement, support and love. The memories I have are like the chain she taught me to crochet—long and beautiful. The circles connecting the chain are everlasting and eternal. With all the love in my heart, dear Grandma, my memories of you will live on forever and my children will know you through them.

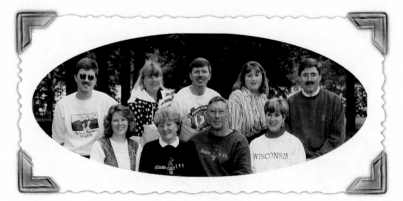

Bella (Ottoson) Girard
Born: July 5, 1933

*I*MAGINE THAT YOUR MOTHER IS DIAGNOSED with Alzheimer's disease and she is only fifty-nine. There is anger, sadness, confusion and anxiety. Now imagine that your maternal grandmother died of Alzheimer's and two of your mother's brothers have also been diagnosed. *That is fear.* This is what we siblings are facing—all seven of us. We have each dealt with this in our own individual way. Some are in denial, some use prayer and for others information is power.

As the years go by, when a sister, brother, or cousin would forget something we'd joke that "they" must be getting it. Then as more years pass, the number touched by this disease in our family has in fact increased, like it has in our nation. The laughter and jokes still continue, but deep down the forgetfulness has taken on a whole new meaning.

We have always admired our mother and father for their devotion and dedication. As adults, we watch with even more admiration as Dad cares for Mom with the same unconditional love she used to give to us.

But we know how this story will end. There is no cure. There are no survivors to be "spokespersons" for this disease like there are for others. So our family has decided to "speak out" while we can. We started a company using our collective talents. Although the four sisters own and operate the company, *Alzheimer's Awareness Source*, it has definitely been a family affair. Dad, brother, aunts and uncles, nieces, nephews and cousins have all helped sell products at the Memory Walks. All of the profits go to the Alzheimer's Association for programs and research and to raise awareness.

This family has truly found a silver lining in a dark cloud. Yet, as I watch my six siblings, and look at my own children I can't help but ask, *"Who will be next?"*

Help find the cure!
Bella's kids
Michigan's Upper Peninsula

Alzheimer's Awareness Source

LIVING WITH DIGNITY, COURAGE AND LOVE

www.alzawareness.com

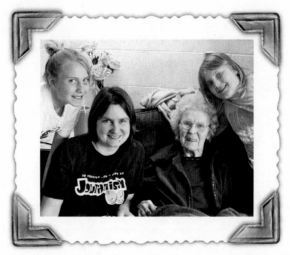

Viola Marjatta (Korvenpaa)Karttunen
August 22, 1913 ~ January 13, 2010

Like Two Berries

Y GRANDMA, VIOLA, IS NINETY-SIX and lives in a nursing home. When I visit her she sometimes doesn't remember me. "Are you one of those people who used to go up the stairs in my house in Green?" she asks.

"Yes, Grandma. I'm Heather, Douglas's daughter."

When I was little, I'd race up the stone path to her house and pull the string on the bell, the eager rings called me to each visit. I used to play upstairs and pull toys & books out from the *koppi* (closet). My favorite book was "Auno and Tauno," about the blond Finnish twins who'd ski to school and get into mischief.

And we'd sauna on Saturdays, pour water on the rocks and listen to it sizzle.

Grandma doesn't remember me that way, as Heather, the little girl racing up a stone path. Each time I see her now she squints to place me, then asks, "Are you the teacher?"

"Yes, Grandma, I teach high school".

"You teach the children." She says. "I think you are a good teacher." And then she smiles and caresses my hand, and we're connected once again.

Grandma likes teachers. When I went to Northern Michigan University, she confided that she had wanted to become a teacher, too. But she got married and had four children. Her life took a different course.

My daughters visit at the nursing home. I wish they could know Grandma Karttunen the way I remember her, usually drying off her hands with a dish towel after pulling out a batch of homemade caramel pecan sticky rolls from the oven, their aroma permeating throughout her home while she apologized, "They didn't' turn out so well this time. They're a little burnt."

But of course everything she made from oatmeal date cookies to turkey dinner, tasted perfectly delicious.

I wish I could preserve Grandma's memories like she preserved the plump raspberries we picked from the patch near the edge of her rain dampened garden. I wish I could open that jar of delectable fruit and release the sweet smell of those summer days in Green to remind her of each sun ripened raspberry, one for each time she made me feel so loved. Grandma had a way of making each child feel special, like you were the most important person in her world. Grandma and me, we were like two berries.

Mostly, I remember walking from her log cabin home that Grandpa built. We'd stroll across the road to Lake Superior's shores. She'd pull out a handmade *huivi* (scarf) to keep the sun off my head. It was red and white gingham, with navy blue anchors and velvet to the touch. At the beach we'd search for driftwood, pick agates and walk barefoot in the sand. The waves lapped onto the shore, hugging our toes before it would recede. Hug and recede. My *huivi* flapped in the breeze, protecting me from harsh rays. Those blue anchors pulled away from the gingham, splashed into the water and secured Grandma and me in our own private world, where the shores of childhood stretch for thousands of miles … and those plump red berries always stay in season.

Heather (Karttunen) Hollands
June 2009/Upper Peninsula Writing Project

Heather is a teacher at Gwinn High School
in Upper Michigan.
"Like Two Berries" is a beautifully compiled video that
can be viewed in its entirety at
http://nwpmichigan.ning.com/video/like-two-berries

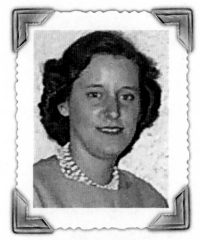

Jean Ann Jackson
January 26, 1931 ~ June 22, 2005

Y PARENTS, NICK AND JEAN ANN were married on June 17, 1948. I am Nick Jr., the oldest of seven children. One of my sisters died as an infant from a birth defect. That seemed to make my family, especially my parents, even closer. We siblings went on to give my parents fourteen grandchildren, and they in turn have blessed us all with twelve great grandkids.

Alzheimer's had been afflicting my mother for several years before my father came to the painful conclusion that he could no longer care for her on his own, and so he put her in a home.

He visited religiously, three times a day and knew almost every resident by name at the time of her death. He exuded a natural, contagious friendliness. My mother's passing was not only a blow to him, but to the other elderly residents who would no longer enjoy a sweet "hello" from Jean Ann's faithful companion.

My mother was always an energetic, outgoing and fun-loving lady. Humor was her survival tactic, but that ALL disappeared with an illness that started slowly but progressed at a shocking rate. Soon after she lost her memory, her ability to speak went, too. Near the end, the fetal position became her only comfort and she was barely able to take nourishment. It was hard seeing her knowing she didn't "see" me back. That's the most difficult thing about losing a loved one to Alzheimer's: You lose them twice— once when they no longer know you, and again upon their death. That was my personal experience and it's painful to share, even after five years. My father has since suffered a stroke. His ability to speak has also been greatly affected. He doesn't talk much about my mother's later years. None of us do. It's hard seeing him suffer, too. But he still knows my name and smiles warmly when I enter the room.

With Love,
Nick Jackson
Peshtigo, Wisconsin

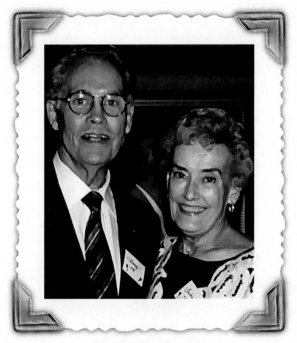

Douglas Van Vechten
March 22, 1920 ~ April 10, 2005

*S*TOIC, BRAVE, WORLD WAR II VETERAN, self-taught piano player, born again Christian, pickled herring and ketchup sandwiches, Lawrence Welk … these are the words that come to mind when I think of my grandfather. He was the type of man that you weren't sure really liked you, even if you were his only grandchild. He liked to attempt to make you laugh with his most distinguished Donald Duck impression, but it didn't generally ever achieve the laughs he was going for.

My grandfather was a California transplant from the Midwest. He followed the American Dream out west. His wife almost immediately landed a job working for some new studio known as Disney while Douglas found work as a backhoe driver. He dug a lake far out past the orange groves. They were digging the lake to build some sort of suburbia away from the Hollywood studios, for the bigwigs. An oasis. A getaway…

When I was young, he would sing us songs and play the piano. They were self-written and self-taught. They were all about God. I used to ask him questions about God. Sometimes, he couldn't answer in a way I understood, but deep down, in my own soul, I knew he had a Faith stronger than anyone else in my life.

I loved visiting with Grandpa and Grandma. They would turn on *The Lawrence Welk Show* and I would dance and prance in Grandma's rhinestone jewels, and occasionally, her real pearls. Grandpa would fix Grandma and me grilled cheese sandwiches for dinner while he put ketchup between two pieces of white bread for himself with a jar of pickled herring on the side. By then, they lived on a lake out in another county, about twenty minutes outside of Burbank, California.

His memory went quick. I think Grandma tried to hide it for a while and I was busy with babies and didn't notice much. Before I knew it, he was living in a care facility. It was one of the best facilities around, since Grandma had a good retirement package. The nurses cared, the doctors cared, the specialists cared. But it wasn't enough. Sometimes he wouldn't know Grandma, or my mom. Occasionally he wouldn't recognize me. But he always knew my boys, or at least it felt that way.

He passed after two years. It felt like more to us. I hope it didn't feel that way to him. The hospital food didn't compare to his ketchup sandwiches and pickled herring.

When I would visit him in the final months, we'd walk the hallways. All of those people had lived "larger than life" in their previous years. Some had been actors. Some had been singers. Some had broken barriers that I will never understand. My Grandfather had fought a war, stolen away another man's fiancée, raised happy children who raised happy children, and given a foundation to us all.

In that little hospital in Calabasas, I was sure that everyone else had good stories, too. As I would look at all of their blank stares, I would say to myself, "I hope they still see the good times."

With Love,
Tracie Madden,
Simi Valley, California

The Acknowledgements before "The Acknowledgements"

I AM TELLING YOU (IN NO UNCERTAIN terms) that if not for the wonderful world of books and the God blessed television, I would have gone insane six months into this "waiting" game. For that, I'd like to send unending thanks to:

Eat, Pray, Love
Elizabeth Gilbert

The Alchemist
Paulo Coelho
(thank you again and again and again)

The Glass Castle
Jeannette Walls

Always Looking Up
(Adventures of an Incurable Optimist)
Michael J. Fox

Sudoku
Any level. Anytime. Anywhere.

Henry VIII
Margaret George

On the Brink of Bliss and Insanity
Lisa Cerasoli
(Hey—I was publishing. I had to read it A LOT.)

"The Twilight Series"
Stephanie Meyer

The Time Traveler's Wife
Audrey Niffenegger
(Got lost in that book twice—amazing!)

Dreams from my Father
Barack Obama

Campingly, Yours
Thomas C. Adler

The Thrillionnaire
Nik Halik

My Sister's Keeper
Jodi Picoult

Home After Dark ... One Man's Memories
Darryl E. Robidoux

Julie & Julia
Julie Powell

Flying For Peanuts
Marty Thompson

Oh, the Places You'll Go
The Cat in the Hat
Fox in Socks
Green Eggs and Ham
One Fish, Two Fish, Red Fish, Blue Fish
Dr. Seuss
(You're a genius. No wonder you made yourself a "Doctor.")

And there are so many more ...

Special Thanks
(when I've been WAY too burnt to flip pages) to:

Oprah
Trading Spaces
Design on a Dime

165

House

Castle

Grey's Anatomy

Private Practice

Life On Mars

Eli Stone

The Starter Wife

Extreme Home Makeover

Weeds

Californication

Curb Your Enthusiasm

True Blood

The United States of Tara

In Therapy

Entourage

Real Time with Bill Maher

Hung

Nurse Jackie

Also,

CNN

Hannah Montana

The Wizard's of Waverly Place

The Suite Life of Zach & Cody

Movie after Movie ON DEMAND

AND...

May God kindly bless every season of *American Idol*, especially seasons two and eight. Season two got my dying father through the winter. He finally had "great vocals" to cry over instead of cancer. It created a whole 'nother diversion for my mother. She developed a much needed obsession with the immensely talented Clay Aiken. She still blames herself for him not claiming the title, stating, "I only voted sixty-three times. I should have kept calling." And Season eight ... what can I say about the best season yet? The talent was awe-inspiring. Adam Lambert's vocal capabilities gave me tingly jolts of life-sustaining adrenaline every Tuesday and Wednesday for months. Plus, Gram could watch this show and almost "get" it. Thank you, *American Idol* for existing. You are loved by every member of my family from age four to eighty-eight.

And thanks to *The Lawrence Welk Show*. You have been mentioned so frequently in this memoir, it's only appropriate to pay homage to a show that bridged the gap and created life-lasting memories for my generation of "grandchildren."

Resources & References

"SPARK"

The Revolutionary New Science of Exercise and the Brain
By
John J. Ratey, MD
with Eric Hagerman

LET'S TALK FANTASTIC: THIS BOOK CREDITS "exercise" through years and years of research and trials as the number one way to boost your memory and sharpen your thinking. Ratey's book is just that: revolutionary. We all know the benefits our body derives from regular exercise, but now there's solid, substantial proof that by conditioning the body, we are actually enhancing our minds. That "high" one feels after a workout isn't just a mood booster, it is literally regenerating your brain, thereby increasing focus and prepping it to obtain and store more knowledge. It's a wonderfully inspiring resource that reminds us to keep our bodies moving and our brains strong. Plus, it instills hope in everyone who lives with the fear that they may become a victim of Alzheimer's or dementia. Now is the time to get proactive, and "exercise" is the way to do it.

"I'm Still Here"
A new philosophy of Alzheimer's Care
By
John Zeisel, Ph.D.

Zeisel's book teaches compassion through creativity. By tapping into the right brain, one can discover that a person suffering from a dementia related illness can be brought out of their shell, over and over again. This can be done through music, art, film and other creative medias. It's a great tool for "filling in the longer days" and for "bonding" with a loved one who otherwise seems lost inside themselves.

"The 36-Hour Day:"
A Family Guide to Caring for Persons with Alzheimer Disease, Related Dementing Illnesses, and Memory Loss in Later Life
By
Nancy L. Mace, M.A. and Peter V. Rabins, M.D., M.P.H.

The main emphasis of this information-packed book with a strong medical tone is that people suffering from these diseases are "ill" not "old." It is also crucial to remember that each person is an individual whose brain stores and processes memories differently than facts. A person's state of emotional well-being plays a major role in how their mind handles the progression of dementia.

Common sense, a sense of humor, imagination and stable environment are emphasized and expounded upon as well.

"What if it's not Alzheimer's?"
A Caregiver's Guide to Dementia
Edited By
Lisa Radin & Gary Radin
Forward by John Trojanowski, M.D. PhD

This book includes vital information on
Frontal Temporal Dementia (FTD)

The ability to remember day-to-day events is critically dependent upon the hippocampus found on the inside of the temporal lobes. The frontal lobe determines our emotional reaction to any given situation. This specific syndrome can create difficulty for a person to maintain any sort of attention span and in conjunction with that, allow them to lose sight of their inhibitions. It can also create a series of cognitive difficulties.

Internet Sites
Web M.D.
Mark Warner's, "Alzheimer's Daily News"
Alzheimer's Awareness Source

The beauty of the internet is it is up-to-date, quick and easily accessible. These sites offer current information in a concise format that is easy for the overwhelmed caregiver to take in without needing to sift through medical jargon and data that simply are not relevant to their particular case.

Keep in mind, they are generalized. That is to say, DO NOT TAKE TO HEART everything you read on the internet.

For example: *The Lap Dog Theory*. There is nothing wrong with this theory. I bet it has eased the burden on many an unsure and exhausted caregiver, and brought genuine joy into the life of the person they are caring for. However, I frantically ran for the "quick fix" without truly regarding the specific person I was caring for ... and it made things tougher.

The Family Doctors

Stephen R. Leonard M.D. of Bellin Health Care has been a Board Registered practicing physician for over thirty years. He has been thorough and informative. There were a series of extensive cognitive tests along with MRIs, ongoing blood tests and regular physical checkups that have been instrumental in helping me with Gram. He also seems to be available for Q & A whenever I phone, even in his off hours (but that's thanks to a small town and a big heart).

It is so important to find a physician that you can trust and feel comfortable enough to rely on for both their knowledge in the field and emotional support. We have been lucky to find that in Doctor Leonard.

Cindy S. Anderson, M.D. of Marquette Internal Medicine & Pediatric Associates, P.C. has been our new doctor since our

Resources & References

recent move to Marquette. She is thorough, informative, patient
and kind. Dr. Anderson and her staff make Gram feel comfortable
and always fit her into their full schedule.

"Take Your Oxygen First:"
*Protecting Your Health & Happiness While Caring for a
Loved One with Memory Loss*
By
Leeza Gibbons

Take Your Oxygen First is a perfect combination of the
pertinent medical facts of dementia-related illnesses mixed with
touching and emotional excerpts from family members. They were
like angels working in perfect sync to help Leeza's Dad survive
the challenges of Alzheimer's while caring for his wife and lifelong companion, Gloria Jean. It a great tool for anyone who needs
fast facts and genuine emotional insight and connection.

Acknowledgements

To all the Guardian Angels in my life. I don't know what I've done to deserve you ... but I'm gonna keep on doing it and hope my thanks will be returned tenfold:

Linda F. Radke of Five Star Publications, Inc., thank you for your insights, genuine dedication and endless, endless enthusiasm. You are one beautiful human being. Thanks to Sue DeFabis (project manager), you are not only always available, but the "collected" to my "frazzled." Paul Howey (editor), you are brilliant, ballsy and kind, which makes you so very cool. And Kris Taft Miller, thank you for another breathtaking cover design. Linda Longmire, your interior design is the perfect, elegant compliment.

Thank you, Sandra Siegal of Siegal Entertainment, Inc. You know you're my "Oprah," and Ken Atchity of Atchity Entertainment, International. You are my Einstein.

Mom,

You know you have been my all-time salvation and my true BFF.
I realize this is my second book ... and still no dedication to you.
My first novel was dedicated to Dad, and this one went to Gram.
So it's like this: If you come down with some really whacked life-
threatening illness, my next book will be all yours.
But please don't do that.
I love you forever.

Pete,

I know some days must feel like a slow, benumbing "death by
Lisa." But without you, I surely would have succumbed to a
quick one. They say Chivalry is dead. Well, I've got a tall, dark,
handsome prototype sitting in my living room to prove otherwise.
Hold on, babe, our honeymoon is out there waiting.

Jazz,

You are my queen. I am forever devoted. When I grow up I hope
to have your spirit, imagination and pizzazz.

Brock,

I did a mighty fine job of bragging you up in the book (if I say so
myself). But listen, dude, you rock. And just as I hope for some
of Jazzy's attributes when I become a big girl, I hope to acquire
your patience and panache.

Rick,

You're the other living proof that real men aren't a thing of history. When the going gets tough, together we've proved it's possible for family to feed upon their strengths. Your wife is a dream and your babe is a miracle. Thanks Jen and Jakey for selflessly loaning me your "man" over and over again for both his brains and his brawn.

And thanks to all my dear friends and relatives who have taken time from their own busy lives to read this manuscript and generously give notes and thoughts and tech support: Kris Leonard, Rose Loeks, Maggie Stang, Fritzi Deichelbor, Laura Dupras, Jeannie Leonard, Spencer Stang, Sean Madden, Cheryl Christ, Marsha Hodges, Valarie Beadle, Shawnee Penachik and Todd Dooley. I cherish you all.

To my "letter writers," thank you for your courage. Your efforts are another example of the beautiful truth behind my mother's most treasured phrase: Life is not Forever ... Love is.

Finally, my sincere thanks to The Alzheimer's Association. Knowing what I know now, is it a coincidence you have the same initials as Alcoholics Anonymous? Just kidding (and just curious). Thank you for supporting my personal experience ... and everyone's experience. My pledge (A buck a book!) is to make you a million dollars. It'll be a small start toward kicking a big disease.

And a very special thanks goes out the to the gorgeous, multi-talented and passionate Leeza Gibbons. I am so fortunate to be joining forces with you and The Leeza Gibbons Memory Foundation in the fight against Alzheimer's Disease. Because of your generosity, insight, humor and heart, you have given this project "wings." I am eternally grateful.

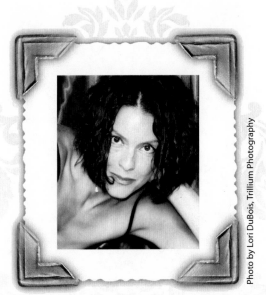

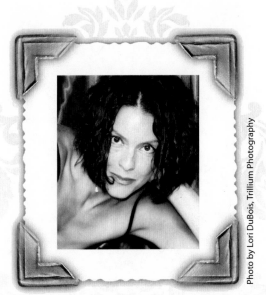
Photo by Lori DuBois, Trillium Photography

Lisa Cerasoli

About The Author

A COMPLISHED ACTOR-TURNED-writer Lisa Cerasoli introduced, "*On the Brink of Bliss and Insanity*" into the world of published fiction in January 2009. In May, it won Honorable Mention at the *San Francisco Book Festival and Midwest Book Review* chose it as "A Top Pick" for New Fiction. "As Nora Jo Fades Away" is Lisa's second book. This surprising memoir bares little resemblance to her debut novel outside of her characteristic in-your-face style. "On the Brink..." is also a screenplay which is currently being shopped in the Hollywood film market, and "Nora Jo..." has been written as a pilot proposal for television under the title *Confessions of a Caregiver.*

Her latest endeavor is working as Senior VP of Development for Five Star Scripts which is an exciting new division of Five Star Publications, www.fivestarscripts.com, where manuscripts are adapted for film and TV.

Lisa and the family moved to Marquette, Michigan in the fall of 2009 for Pete's job. Brock travels between parents and is crazy busy being fifteen and playing varsity basketball for Kingsford High School. Jazz loves school and the YMCA. G.G. loves "Jazz," so she gets her "exercise" too, which has made her forget she's a fan of "sitting and drinking." The upside to Alzheimer's? Gram has forgotten she likes "the beer."

More information about this author can be found on the Five Star site as well as www.LisaCerasoli.com. And you can leave questions and comments for Lisa at www.AsNoraJoFadesAway. com where you will also find up-to-date news about book sales, funds raised for the Alzheimer's Association, this disease, Nora Jo and the family.

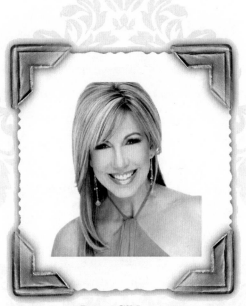

Leeza Gibbons

About Leeza

HE SPECTRUM OF LEEZA GIBBONS' career in entertainment and news media combined with her stunning "hands on" advocacy for healthcare, patients and caregivers is diverse and impressive. Leeza's on-camera hosting dominance in entertainment news and talk show arenas range from the most popular entertainment news show in history, *Entertainment Tonight* to TV news magazine *Extra.* For six years she was producer and host of the eponymous *Leeza* - the Emmy award winning daytime show covering pop-culture, beauty, medical and social issues. Her radio show, *Hollywood Confidential* reaches over 3.5 million listeners in the United States and Canada and her direct response *Sheer Cover* beauty and cosmetics infomercial show is in its 7th year with worldwide viewership in the tens of millions.

Leeza's compassion, inspiration and commitment to her continual education of self and others, is a special gift potentiated by her listening and communication skills honed as a mother, journalist and humanitarian. It was her family's experience with Leeza's mother and grandmother that inspired her to create *The Leeza Gibbons Memory Foundation* (a 501c3 non-profit) and its signature program, *Leeza's Place*. Now there are eight Leeza's Place locations nationwide offering free services for caregivers of loved ones with any chronic illness or disease. She also wrote a book about her personal experience called *Take Your Oxygen First: Caring for Yourself while Caring for Someone with Memory Loss*, which was just named one of the best consumer health books in the marketplace from *Library Journal*, with additional kudos from *Publishers Weekly*.

Leeza found a natural outlet on the Lifetime Series, *Health Corner*, a weekly TV magazine show focusing on providing viewers with information on health, wellness and prevention and the latest discoveries in the health field. During the course of almost 100 episodes of the *Lifetime* series, *What Should You Do?* Leeza empowered viewers with help and advice for dealing with life-threatening emergencies. She also is the founder and creator of *Sheer Inspiration Life Coaching*, a web based business offering one-on-one access to help individuals reclaim, reinvent or enhance their lives.

Numerous guest appearances on *Larry King Live, Good*

Morning America, *Oprah*, *The Today Show*, *Donny Duestch* and *The View* have all centered around her role as a social entrepreneur. Most recently she was named one of the "Ten Who Make a Difference" by *AARP* being called the "Voice of the Caregiver." Leeza has been on the board of the *Alzheimer's Association* for over a decade, as well as a two decade commitment to the celebrity panel of the *American Red Cross*. She is also one of California Governor Arnold Schwarzenegger's appointees to the *Independent Citizen's Oversight Committee*, the governing board of the *California Institute of Regenerative Medicine*.

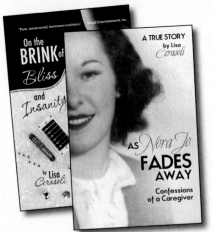

As Nora Jo Fades Away

Order Form

After luring us through her debut novel, *On the Brink of Bliss and Insanity* with stark wit and mad fascinating charaters, Lisa Cerasoli surprises us with her second book–the heartfelt true story of life with h ailing Grandmother. remaining loyal to the "raw truth trait" that exemplifies her writing style, *As Nora Jo Fades Away* will make your heart and mind wrestle, as Cerasoli's does, with concepts like logic vs. love, laughter vs. tears, Heaven and Hell.

ITEM	QTY	Unit Price	TOTAL
Nora Jo Fades Away		$15.95	
On the Brink of Bliss and Insanity		$15.95	
➤➤➤➤➤➤➤➤➤➤➤➤➤➤➤➤➤➤ Subtotal			
* 7.8% sales tax – on all orders originating in Arizona.		*Tax	
* $8.00 or 10% of the total order – whichever is greater. Ground shipping. Allow 1 to 2 weeks for delivery.		*Shipping	
Mail form to: Five Star Publications, PO Box 6698, Chandler, AZ 85246-6698		TOTAL	

NAME:

ADDRESS:

CITY, STATE, ZIP:

DAYTIME PHONE: FAX:

EMAIL:

Method of Payment:
❑VISA ❑Master Card ❑Discover Card ❑American Express

▲ account number   ▲ expiration date

▲ signature   ▲ 3-4 digit security numbe

❑ Yes, please send me a Five Star Publications catalog.
❑ Send me info about the co-authors speaking at my event.
How were you referred to Five Star Publications?
❑ Friend ❑ Internet ❑ Book Show ❑ Other

Five Star Publications
Twenty-Five Year Anniversary 1985-2010

P.O. Box 6698 • Chandler, AZ 85246-66
(480) 940-8182 866-471-0777 Fax: (480) 940-87
info@FiveStarPublications.com www.FiveStarPublications.cc

Got a Memory? Jot it Down